STOP ARTHRITIS

****

HOW I DEFEATED IT NATURALLY

****

MY PROGRAM REVEALED

****

ALAN SCHLINES

"Stop Arthritis: My Program Revealed," by Alan Schlines. ISBN 1-58939-426-7.

Published 2003 by Virtualbookworm.com Publishing Inc., P.O. Box 9949, College Station, TX , 77842, US. ©2003 Alan Schlines. All rights reserved. No part of this publication may be reproduced, stored in a retrieval system, or transmitted in any form or by any means, electronic, mechanical, recording or otherwise, without the prior written permission of Alan Schlines.

Manufactured in the United States of America.

Acknowledgments

I would like to extend my deepest gratitude to my parents and family for their support, patience and understanding throughout this entire program. There were many ups and downs, but together we conquered it. Also, I would like to thank Dr. Marcus Ettinger, Dr. Lis Baird, Gary Richer, and Dr. Terry Pfau for their guidance. Without their superior knowledge, wisdom, and overall caring personalities, my success would not have been possible. Also I would like to thank Brad Cantrell for having an open mind and the insightfulness to introduce me to Dr. Baird. Without this introduction, my program would have been incomplete. And finally I would like to thank God for helping me through some of the most difficult times of my life.

Important Note

The material in this book is for informational purposes only. It is not intended to serve as a prescription for you, or to replace the advice of your medical doctor. Please discuss all aspects of this book with your physician before beginning the program. If you have any medical conditions, or are taking any prescription or nonprescription medications, see your physician before beginning the program or altering or discontinuing your use of medication.

Contents

Preface...7
Foreword 10
1. My First Symptoms 14
2. Going to the Doctor -- The Diagnosis.................................19
3. Following the Doctor's Orders or Not 23
4. Dr. Marcus Ettinger -- The Gerson Program Started.........30
    Gerson Program 31
    Detoxification Program...36
    Colon Program (Enemas)..40
    Juicing Program 43
    Sauna Program (Hyperthermia) 45
5. Dr. Lis Baird -- Kinesiology and Herbology Explored 48
    Benefits of Chiropractic..50
    Applied Kinesiology...51
    Herbology 53
6. Gary Richer -- The Live Cell King 63
    Live Cell Analysis 64
    Iris Analysis (Iridology) 68
    Cycle Detoxification Program 71
7. Dr. Terry Pfau -- Homeopathic Help from Las Vegas.........73
    Homeopathic Program 74
8. Other Natural Supplements -- Immune System Boosters...........78
9. Other Programs Learned and Explained 96
10. Arthritis Stopped: My Immune System Wins 104
    Immune System..106
    Air (Oxygen)..108
    Water 110
    Digestion 113
    Exercise 119
    Sleep..121
    Attitude and Emotions...122
11. Food Choices -- What's Good, What's Bad 125

Standard American Diet (SAD)..126
Recommended Dietary Allowances vs. Optimum Dietary
Allowances...130
Food Comparisons..133
Long-Term Health 149
The Food Commandments 153
My 10 Worst Foods List 154
Organic Foods vs. Non-Organic Foods....................159
Cooking Methods...160
Natural Hygiene Products...161
Cigarette Smoking 163
12. Drugs vs. Nature -- Which is Safer? 169
Food and Drug Administration (FDA) 172
Safety Statistics Revealed..175
13. Health vs. Wealth -- The Money Factor 169
Teach Health or Teach Wealth? 185
Shocking Health Statistics...188
Are We the Healthiest Country?................................190
14. Summary: Together We Can Defeat It.....................194
Endnotes...198

Preface

In 1968, it was estimated that 13 million Americans suffered
from arthritis. Today, over 35 years later, estimates are that
over 70 million Americans suffer from this crippling disease. This equates to 1 out every 4 persons in America that will
eventually succumb to the disease. With this number growing at
an alarming rate, obviously something is terribly wrong with the
approach that the medical establishment has taken towards arthritis. The medical approach suggests that you should take the prescribed medicine, hope that it helps with the pain, have surgery
when needed, and learn to live with it. *There is no true hope
given to the patient, since the medical establishment states that
there is no cure.* If you or your loved ones currently have arthritis, then you know that having no hope is extremely disheartening. Ten years ago, I was one of these patients that were given no
hope. But instead of letting arthritis control my life and being
forced to learn to live with the pain, I decided to take control of
my own life. I decided that there had to be a better way. In *Stop
Arthritis*, I will show you that there is a better way and that you
don't have to live with this crippling disease any longer.

Over the last fifty years, our society has been trained by
the medical establishment that if you are diagnosed with arthritis,
you should go to the doctor and take the prescribed medications.
This seems like the logical thing to do, since medical doctors are
highly trained professionals. Unfortunately, medical doctors are
trained to treat diseases with drugs, not by using natural methods.
In their four or more years of medical school they are taught very
little, if any at all, about nutrition, natural methods, and their
benefits to the body. Instead, they are taught to pinpoint the area
of the disease and then treat it with a prescription drug. But, the
problem with this approach is that drugs only treat the symptoms

that you are having and will never treat the underlying problem, which is the disease in itself. It is only these natural methods that will strengthen your immune system so that your body can rise up and defeat the disease once and for all. I will show you the programs that are necessary to permanently defeat arthritis and also explain how these programs will improve your overall health.

I am not a medical doctor. This is a key advantage to you for several reasons. First, I will explain my true story on how I was struck down with incurable arthritis. I will walk you step-by-step through my entire program, including: my first symptoms, my diagnosis, my decision to go with the natural approach, meeting the natural doctors, learning and using their programs, and finally defeating arthritis for good. In addition, I will explain in detail all the research I have accumulated over the last ten years regarding different subjects including: vitamins, herbs, juicing, detoxification, immune system strengthening, healthy food choices, the safety of vitamins versus drugs, and the problems with the overall health of our country today. *Another key advantage is that this book is based on facts.* I have gathered research from over 100 different types of professionals including M.D.'s, Ph.D.'s, Ph.N.'s, N.D.'s, D.C.'s, D.O.'s, R.N.'s, D.D.S.'s, and M.H.A's, to name just a few. This research comes from highly prestigious medical institutions such as UCLA, Harvard, Yale, U.C. Berkeley, B.Y.U., Cornell, Tufts, Arizona State, Loma Linda, etc... so obviously it can be trusted. So if your doctor or anyone else tells you that defeating arthritis is "not proven", or "no research has been done", or "you need to take prescription drugs," please do not listen to them. Instead, show them this book, because it contains all the research and proof that is needed to stop arthritis.

This book is directed towards the average layman. I have described the programs that I used in an easy-to-follow format, in hopes that you make the decision to use the same approach. Modern medicine has failed in its drug approach towards arthritis, since they state it is an incurable disease. I, on the other hand, have not failed and believe just the opposite about this crippling disease. As of this writing, I have been pain-free for over ten years. At my lowest point my body was attacking my joints at an increasingly rapid pace, leaving a few of my joints deformed. At one point I couldn't walk for over a month and a half, and was almost wheelchair bound. By using the natural programs in this book, along with some discipline and patience, I was able to stop my arthritis and enjoy a pain-free life once again. My full intention of this book is to provide you with enough medical facts and research to make it an easy decision for you to go with the natural approach. I think it is ridiculous to see so many lives ruined by this agonizing disease. Each and every one of the 70 million-plus arthritis sufferers out there has endured long enough with the pain and suffering. *There is a better way and it's called the natural way.* The information is now at your fingertips, giving you the power to change your life forever. Do not sit on the sidelines, but take action and take control of your life today!

To Your Health,
Alan Schlines
March, 2003

Foreword

Dictionaries have many definitions for the word "responsible". The first one fits what I feel I do as a doctor: "legally or ethically accountable for the welfare of another." When I graduated from Chiropractic College, I swore an oath to be responsible for anyone who seeks my care, and I feel I have never violated that oath. There are two other definitions that fit how I act in my personal life and how others, if responsible, should act. *1) "Involving personal accountability or ability to act without guidance or superior authority." 2) "Capable of making moral or rational decisions on one's own, therefore answerable for one's behavior."* The reason I bring this up is because the word responsible has been, I feel, year after year gradually losing its meaning. I have been noticing the *obvious* effects of this in my practice and in my surroundings for some time.

Today, I feel most people who are experiencing health-related problems are either doing nothing (no responsibility) or are placing total responsibility on the doctor, whether it's getting their health back or maintaining it at a certain level. Examples: if you have high "this" or low "that", take a drug. If it's clogged or malfunctioning, remove it. If it's too fast or too slow, take another drug. If you think there may be a problem now or in the future but aren't sure yet, take a drug just to be on the safe side. This complacent attitude our culture has developed is extremely dangerous, and has contributed to hundreds of thousands of needless deaths, surgeries, hospitalizations, and billions of dollars a year spent on medications. *Medications only treat symptoms, while masking the underlying condition or disease state.* Geneticists (doctors who study and research our genetic makeup, DNA, etc...) state that we reach our genetic potential around 30-35 years of age. This means that we are as good as we are ever going to be at that age. After that, our bodies start to deteriorate. Some of us go through this process very slowly, while others do so quite rapidly. The rate of this deterioration depends slightly on genetics, and predominately on *responsibility*. It's not the responsibility of doctors, family and friends, Richard Simmons or Jenny Craig. *It's your responsibility!*

Taking responsibility for your health has four components: First, there is *education*. Educate yourself on diet, anatomy, exercise, health or anything that may benefit you in living longer and healthier. Second is *nutrition*. Eat to support every cell of your body, not just for the taste or because it's a "good deal". Third is *exercise*. If you don't move it or use it, you will lose it! Nothing can be truer. The surest way to get osteoporosis, arthritis, sore joints, weak muscles and tendons or a slow metabolism is by not exercising. Fourth is *changing your environment*. If you're in a place that you don't want to be because it's not aesthetically pleasing, the people are negative toward you or unethical behavior is occurring, etc...get out! These four components, when not actively followed, have been proven to weaken our immune system by placing undue negative stress on us.

The four components for taking responsibility of your health may seem obvious to some, and to others may seem as foreign as learning Chinese. For those of you who are acting responsibly toward your health, *I validate your effort.* For those of you who believe your body will run forever without any needed adjustment to your present condition, or believe that all the aches and pains, stiffness, inability to eat the foods you did when you were younger, high blood pressure, high cholesterol and increased weight are just signs of getting older and that it's "inevitable", you are either wrong or just misinformed.

Poor health equals "irresponsibility". You, yourself, have personally helped create this condition by lack of following the above four components to health. It's not to late too change your present condition. Recognizing that a problem exists, and also recognizing that a positive change needs to occur is all that is required.

Alan Schlines did. Alan is no longer imprisoned by a death sentence of incurable autoimmune arthritis. The medical establishment was the judge that initially sentenced him and threw away the key. Responsibility was the power that set him free. *Alan's book can be your first step to a new and better you.*

P.S. The words "responsible" and "responsibility" are two words I feel we need to pay serious attention to. Our culture has lost personal accountability for everything – *It's not my fault!* These four words are destroying our civilization: morally, ethically, spiritually and physically. If each one of us would take responsibility for our own little piece of the universe, the impact it would have on the big picture would be more significant than can be imagined. *Don't just think about this, do something about it!*

Sincerely,
Marcus Stewart Ettinger B.Sc., D.C.
March 2003

STOP ARTHRITIS

1

My First Symptoms

It all started in the month of October of 1992, when I noticed my first symptoms of pain. I was twenty-four years old and working full-time at a sporting goods store during the day, and going to school at night. Just a few months earlier, I had completed a basketball scholarship from Chapman University, but I was still enrolled in two classes I needed to graduate with a business degree. I was excited that my college career was almost over and I would be able to use my new diploma to move on to bigger and better things. I was ready to go out into the business world to build a lucrative career. But what happened to me next changed my plans extensively, and was the type of life-changing event that I wouldn't forget for the rest of my life.

One day, I was at the sporting goods store working my normal shift when all of a sudden I felt a small pain in the joint of the first toe on my right foot. I didn't think it was a big deal at the time, and thought it could have been that I stepped on it wrong during a basketball game, or that I worked out too hard at the gym. But after a few days the pain wasn't going away like most other aches I'd had; it just seemed to linger. After about a week of this annoying pain, I noticed another painful spot, but this time it was in my right heel. So I decided that every day after work I would ice my right foot to see if this might help with the pain and swelling. I knew that icing my ankles after basketball practice helped, so naturally I gave this a try. I tried it for about a week and it didn't seem to help much, so I started taking Advil thinking this would alleviate the pain. But within one month the pain and swelling just grew worse and it had also moved into three of the toes on my right foot. The pain in my heel had reached the point where I was limping at work, and every step was excruciating. I tried adding shoe inserts for extra padding, but had no success with this either. My limping was very obvious to my co-workers and they knew that something was wrong. They asked me if everything was okay, but I couldn't give them a definite answer. I had no idea as to what was causing me so much pain. I thought it might be from standing at work for eight hours a day, but I wasn't sure. I needed to find an answer because, as everyone knows, living in pain is miserable.

So I decided to visit the head athletic trainer back at my university. I still had a good relationship with him, since just a few months earlier I was in the training room every day for basketball practice. At this point my right toes had improved significantly, so I only mentioned the pain in my right heel. I explained that when I woke up in the morning the pain was at its worst. Putting my right foot down for the first time was incredibly painful, and it felt like all the muscles had tightened up and were trying to stretch out. He examined me and his expert opinion was that it was plantar fasciitis. I had no idea what that was, so he further explained that plantar fasciitis, by definition, is a heel spur that often leads to pain from standing too long, no arch support, or a sudden increase in activity. He recommended that I should stay off my feet as much as possible for a couple of weeks, and to try taping them for extra support. He also recommended that I should ice my foot and take an over-the-counter pain medication, which I was already doing. So I left the training room feeling more confident and went home and did what the trainer recommended.

It was now December of 1992, and I only had one month left to graduate with my business degree. Much to my surprise, I was still experiencing pain and swelling in my right foot. I was in too much pain to continue working at the sporting goods store so I turned in my resignation. I limped to my two night classes with a grimace of pain on my face and proceeded to graduate. I didn't have the big celebration that I had always dreamed about for just graduating from a major university, because I was in too much pain to enjoy it. Every step I took felt like I was getting a needle injected into my heel. I remember going out partying with my friends to try to celebrate my graduation, but it always ended up not being much of a party. We would be drinking and dancing and having a good time, but after a few short hours I could barely limp back to my car because my heel was throbbing with pain. The alcohol seemed to help the pain while I was partying, but in the morning it was always much worse. I continued to party with my friends on several more occasions in hopes of forgetting about my current health situation, but it didn't help. Who was I trying to fool? I had been in pain for two months now and was very depressed. I remember thinking to myself, *"What is going on with my body? I am too young to be in this much pain!"*

So it was on to a new year, 1993, and my future looked bleak with my right foot in its current condition. I had a new business degree in hand, but I was held back because of my foot. I was living with my parents, so luckily I didn't have to worry about rent. For the next two months I didn't work as I waited for the pain to go away. As time went by it seemed to gradually improve, and this was probably because I was off my feet most of the time. With the pain diminishing, I had a new level of confidence and decided to find another job. This time I had to find employment in which I wasn't standing all day like the sporting goods store. In the back of my mind I was worried that if I found another job in which I was standing, the pain would come right back. So after a short search, I was fortunate to find a new job with a rental car company. I was under the impression that I wouldn't be standing up much of the time, so I had high hopes.

It was now March of 1993, and I began working again. My new manager told me that most of my duties would be driving to pick up and drop off the customers, so I knew I would be off my feet most of the time. My other duty would be to occasionally work at the counter helping customers. For the first month everything seemed perfect. I had extra padding in my shoes, so when I did have to stand at the counter it didn't really bother me. But after a month of working that same schedule, things suddenly changed. They wanted me to stay at the counter full-time, putting an end to my pickup and delivery time. Oh well, my plan just flew out the window, and now I was back to standing all day at work. Within one week the pain came rushing back into my right heel and toes, and I was back to square one. I asked my manager if I could put a stool behind the counter to rest my feet but he denied me, with the reason being that it wasn't professional to be sitting when the customers came in the front door. I hesitantly agreed with him and continued to stand all day long. Just as I thought, the pain grew worse and worse. I decided this job just wasn't working out either, so I handed in another resignation. The pain was just too much to bear. I was extremely frustrated, confused, and even scared. What was going on with my body, and why would the pain not subside?

May of 1993 was here, and my career as a rental car agent had only lasted a brief two months. It was back to waiting at home and hoping for the pain to disappear. It had now been approximately five months with this on-and-off pain in my right foot. I hadn't been to a doctor up to this point, because the pain would come and go as if it were trying to trick me. I would have good days in which there would be no pain, and others where it was unbearable. Plus, I was stubborn and really didn't like going to doctors that much. I was also having lower back pain, and my family and I thought that a possible cause of the pain in my right foot might be related to my back. We thought I might have pinched nerves in my lower back, causing pain signals to be sent to my foot. So my mother recommended that I go see a local chiropractor that she had been a patient of over the last few years. She always experienced great results with him, so we decided this would be a great place to begin. It was now time to go meet the chiropractor.

The first visit felt like any other chiropractor I had been to in the past. He performed the normal back adjustments and placed me on one of those heated massage tables. While it was very relaxing and my back felt amazing, it didn't seem to do much for my heel and toe pain. Over the next couple of weeks, I returned to the chiropractor for three or four more adjustments. I felt it wasn't helping my condition, so I decided to stop going. With that decision being made, in hindsight, I probably didn't give him a fair chance to correctly diagnose my condition (I will

explain why in chapter 3). After another week at home, unbe-
lievably I noticed another pain and this time it was in my left ankle. I was stunned because my right toes were already swollen
and painful, my right heel had needle-like pain, my lower back
ached, and now this. It was in the lower portion of my left ankle
and the skin was red, swollen, and hot to the touch, just like my
right toes. I was asking myself "What could be next?" Well, I
probably shouldn't have asked that question, because over the
next couple of days I noticed that my sacroiliac joints (hip area),
lower ribs and spine, and of all things my left pinkie, were all becoming stiff and painful.

My symptoms were increasing very quickly now and
were extremely intense. *I felt like my body was blowing up!* I was
taking ten to twelve Advil a day and icing both feet to try to keep
the swelling down. I wasn't sleeping well and would wake up
several times during the night with throbbing pain in my toes,
heel, ankle, hips, and lower back. I could feel the pain with each
pulse of my blood, rushing to these "hot spots". And as if the
night wasn't bad enough, when I finally did wake up in the morning it was exceedingly worse. I had never been in so much pain in
my life. Trying to stand up and make my way to the bathroom
was ridiculous. First, I had to try to stretch out my toes and ankles. Then I would sit up and try to stretch out my lower back and
lastly I would try to gently put one foot down at a time. Standing
up for the first time was miserable because my lower back was so
stiff, and with my body weight bearing down on my feet, it was
excruciating. I remember taking really long, hot showers because
that seemed like the only thing that would loosen my body up and
help with the pain. I felt like a ninety-year-old man, yet I was just
twenty-five years old. My body was breaking down and it had
only been six months since my first symptoms. It was at this
point in my life that I realized that there was something terribly
wrong with my body; it felt like it was attacking itself. It was
evident that I needed to go see a doctor as quickly as possible.

2

Going to the Doctor
The Diagnosis

It was time to find out the problem with my body and why it felt like it was attacking itself. I scheduled an appointment with an orthopedic surgeon, since they are trained to deal with problems of the bones and joints. I figured it would be the best place to start. When I first walked in for my appointment, I clearly remember how much pain I was in and how tough it was just to enter the office. I filled out all the necessary paperwork and waited for the doctor to call my name. When they called my name I walked into the exam room and shook the doctor's hand. I will never forget the look on his face when he saw my right shoe. I was wearing an old pair of high-top basketball shoes, and I had cut holes in the sides and top so that the shoe would stretch out. I did this so my swollen right foot could fit into it. He was astonished at how swollen it was, but I told him I had been constantly icing it without any success. He than proceeded to take some x-rays of my back, hips, ankles, and feet. He also took some blood samples and asked me some general questions. When he was done with the exam he told me to call back in about a week to find out the results of the x-rays and blood work.

I anxiously waited the entire week. It was one of the longest weeks of my life, because I was afraid of what the results might reveal. I was fearful of the unknown. Fear is a strange emotion, because it can make a situation much worse than it actually is by letting your imagination run wild. Often times when we face difficult situations, we let our imaginations picture the worst possible scenario. I was trying my hardest to keep my vision clear of all fearful thoughts. So at this point I still had no idea what was wrong with my body, just that it hurt like hell. I didn't sleep well at all that week because of the pain and fear I was going through. Finally, the week was over and I nervously called the doctor's office to find out the test results. The doctor didn't tell me much over the phone, but he did insist that I make an appointment with one of his colleagues, who was a rheumatoid arthritis specialist. So with that piece of news, all I knew at this point was that it must be some kind of arthritis. I reluctantly made this next appointment for a few days later and anxiously waited once again.

A few days went by and it was time to go see this rheumatologist. He was a highly acclaimed doctor at a well-respected hospital, so I had the utmost confidence in the situation. I had a morning appointment and was extremely nervous to go see this doctor, due to what the test results might reveal. I remember putting on my walkman headphones in my room and blasting the music to try to get pumped up and gain enough confidence to go see him. I listened to my music for a few minutes and decided it was time to go face reality. So my father drove me down to my appointment. We went into the doctor's office to find out more details of my results from my previous visit to the orthopedic doctor. He called my name, and the time had come to see my test results that possibly could alter my entire future. I changed into the little robe that you have to wear and gingerly sat down on the doctor's table. I was not only nervous, but also very curious as to what had been causing me so much pain over the last six months of my life. The doctor had my x-rays up on the wall so we could view the results together. He clearly pinpointed spots on my pelvis, ankle, and toes that showed joint damage, and also the areas where my spine was slowly fusing together. *I couldn't believe what was happening to my body!* He then went over my blood work and explained that I had tested positive for HLA-B27, a genetic marker that strongly links a person to certain forms of arthritis. Next, he had me do some bending and stretching tests to determine my level of flexibility and maneuvered some of my joints around to find out my range of motion. And then the next four words that came out of his mouth were words that would change my life forever: *"You Have Incurable Arthritis!"*

I was extremely frightened. Of course I had heard of arthritis before but I wasn't quite sure what he meant by incurable. So he proceeded to explain exactly what incurable (autoimmune) forms of arthritis were and how they differed from other forms of arthritis. He told me the two forms I had were Ankylosing Spondylitis (AS) and Reiter's Syndrome. I thought to myself, "Great, not only do I have arthritis, but I have two types of incurable arthritis." He said that I would have to go on medication immediately, and would probably be on medication for the rest of my life, because there was no cure for arthritis. The only hope was learning to cope with it. I remember that sentence very clearly… *"No hope, just cope!"* It ran through my head over and over: no hope, just cope, no hope, just cope. That just seemed like such an overwhelming concept, to have no hope in a situation like this. So he began writing out a prescription and handed me some sample medication, along with a few pamphlets on arthritis. He put me on a medication called Naprosyn and told me to take it once in the morning and once again at night, and that would help control the pain and inflammation. It would help me live a better life. He scheduled another appointment for me to come back in about a month to see how my body was responding to the medication. And that was it. My future had been decided in a thirty-minute office visit. I had incurable arthritis, and now I had to learn to cope with it because there was no cure. I slowly limped out of the office with my father and depressingly told him the doctor's diagnosis. As we drove home we sat in dead silence. *Life felt hopeless!*

I was in complete shock at this point. I had just graduated from college a few months earlier on a basketball scholarship, and thought I was in the best shape of my life. I considered myself to be a great athlete. I was 6'6", 215 lbs., and my body fat level was a low 7%. My vertical leap was about 32 inches, and I could dunk a basketball with ease. In the weight room I was benching 275 lbs., squatting 315, and doing bicep curls with 60 lb. dumbbells. Out on the track for basketball conditioning we were running 220's and 440's, and had to run the mile in under 6:00 minutes. I had been an athlete my whole life. I started playing sports at the age of six. I played various sports like basketball, football, baseball, track, and cross-country all through elementary school, junior high, and high school. I continued playing basketball at junior college, and then received a basketball scholarship to Chapman University. My room was filled with various trophies and awards from different championships. The reason I am telling you this is to illustrate the type of person that I was, and the shape that I was in. Yet within just six short months, my body had completely backfired and I was crippled and could barely walk. I had two forms of incurable arthritis and only one option, and that was to listen to the doctor. I had to take my medication and learn to cope with it. I thought arthritis was something that happened to older people, not a twenty-five year old in almost perfect physical shape. Arthritis doesn't care who it attacks, young or old, in great shape or not. What a life-changing situation I was going through. I was wishing this were all a big nightmare, and when I awoke it would all be back to normal. But it wasn't; I had to face reality and the fact that my life was going to be different from this point forward.

3

Following the Doctor's Orders or Not?

The diagnosis had been given, and six months of complete uncertainty were over. I had incurable arthritis and had to learn to live with it. There was some relief in finding out what was so drastically affecting my body, and having a specific medication for the pain and swelling. My fear had been slightly subdued because the doctor pinpointed what had been causing me so much pain. But there were those four specific words that came out of the doctor's mouth that still stood out in my mind. I couldn't stop thinking about the phrase he said: *"no hope, just cope."* It just didn't feel right to me - that as great as the United States is in the field of medicine, there was no cure for this crippling disease and that I just had to cope with it for the rest of my life. Wasn't America supposed to be the greatest in the medical field? Aren't American doctors supposed to be the best? Oh well, the doctor gave me my diagnosis and it was time for me to get on with my life, take my medication, and go start a new career.

Sometimes looking for a new job is more frustrating than the job itself. Luckily, at that time my father had a friend working for a computer company that had an open position as a marketing assistant. This fit in perfectly with my business degree, so I decided to give it a shot. I went in for the interview and all went well. I started work immediately, and everything seemed to be going just fine in my life. I was taking my medication twice a day, once in the morning and again once at night, just like the doctor ordered. The pain in my heel, ankle, toes, and lower back slowly improved, and life seemed bearable for a change. The mornings that were so painful before, now were at least manageable. I felt like a normal person for a change. While working for this computer company, I would go to all the local libraries and bookstores in my spare time to research and gain as much knowledge about this incurable disease as I could. They all seemed to say the same thing the doctor told me. Most of these books would give a definition of what arthritis is, explain the diagnosis process, tell you what medications to take, and explain ways of coping with it in the future. I looked back at the last six months of my life and said to myself, "That's exactly how it happened in my case." I felt comfortable with my situation and decided to continue to follow the doctor's orders of taking the prescribed medication.

The next week, my mom returned from her regular chiropractor visit and had some very interesting news for me. When she was finishing with her treatment, the doctor kindly asked her how I was doing, and she explained to him that we just found out about a month ago that I had incurable arthritis. The doctor seemed interested, and wanted to know what I was going to do about it. She explained to him that I was following the rheumatologist's orders and taking the medication as directed, and was learning to cope with it. He seemed very disturbed by this and insisted that I immediately make an appointment to come down and talk with him. When my mom told me that he wanted to see me, I wasn't all that excited, because just a few months earlier I had been to the orthopedic doctor, the rheumatologist, and I didn't feel like seeing another doctor. I was doctored out, so to speak. Plus, I had already seen this chiropractor just a few months before, and wasn't sure what he could do differently now that would help me. I was on doctor's orders to take my medication, and it seemed to be working for me, so that's what I was going to do.

My mom insisted, and said that the chiropractor might have a better way of dealing with arthritis and wanted to explain it to me in more detail. When I heard those words, *"a better way to deal with arthritis"*, it really peaked my curiosity. I had come up empty while reading the fifteen or so arthritis books at the libraries and bookstores, so I thought the chiropractor might reveal something new. I thought it would be worth my while to at least go down and listen to him. Lucky for me, my mom was being persistent for me to go back to him. She must have had some kind of divine intervention to push me the way she did. You know what they say about mother's intuition. If I had decided to not go back to see him, that would have been the worst decision I've ever made in my life. I owe a heartfelt thanks to my mom for insisting that I go back.

So I made an appointment to go see the chiropractor again in anticipation of learning a better way to deal with this painful arthritis. I went into his office, and it was much different this time around. He seemed very excited to see me, I guess in anticipation of what he was about to reveal to me. Instead of going into the normal room for my adjustment and massage like I did previously, this time he took me into his private office and sat me down next to him at his desk. He asked me how I was feeling. I explained that I was taking the medication as prescribed, and that it was helping with the pain and inflammation. I had brought my paperwork from my rheumatologist, and showed him the blood work and overall diagnosis (Ankylosing Spondylitis and Reiter's Syndrome). He didn't seem all that interested in the results, which surprised me at first, but I could tell he was more excited about a book he was holding in his hand. I was curious at this point what the book was, and that's when my world began to change. He put the book down in front of me, and the title immediately jumped out at me, *"A Cancer Therapy- Results of Fifty Cases"* by Max Gerson, M.D. I was startled that the title was in reference to cancer. I looked up at the doctor and told him, *"I don't have cancer, I have arthritis"*. He seemed to smile, knowing that he was about to open my eyes to a whole new way of thinking.

This is where it gets interesting. He began explaining to me about the immune system and how it doesn't matter if it is arthritis, cancer, heart disease, stroke, high blood pressure, etc.

He explained that any and all degenerative-type illnesses could be helped, or even stopped, by strengthening the immune system. He further explained that Dr. Max Gerson might be one of the boldest and brightest men of our times to approach health and the human body as he did. He was very specific about the Gerson program, and how it focused on detoxification of the entire system, proper nutrition, and other complimentary programs (I will describe these all in great detail later). We sat and talked for over an hour about the immune system, and how the body can heal itself if given the right healing environment. He said he would let me borrow the book so I could get a better understanding of it and to make sure it made sense to me. He wanted to make sure that I was comfortable with this type of natural program. I was really interested and wanted to go home and read it as quickly as possible, but I also told him I would have to talk it over with the rheumatologist to see what he thought of the program.

So I went home, and over the next couple of days I read the entire book and really focused on the specific programs that the fifty cancer patients all used to heal themselves, *naturally*. It was a unique approach that focused on juicing organic vegetables, detoxifying the body, and using natural, organic foods. *It focused on the body's number one priority in life, which is to survive and overcome diseases.* The surprising thing is that not only did Dr. Max Gerson's program cure cancer, it also cured things like high blood pressure, asthma, migraines, tuberculosis, skin diseases, diabetes, and of course, arthritis. Many of these conditions are considered incurable. This seemed absolutely amazing to me! I knew my next appointment with my rheumatologist was about a week away, so this gave me time to do some extra research. My research this time was much different. Instead of looking up books on arthritis, I was looking up books on topics such as the immune system, detoxification, natural health, and holistic programs. I found a few books that backed up Dr. Gerson's ideas of a natural approach towards disease. These new ideas seemed much more logical to me. It made more sense than taking medication the rest of my life and just coping with the pain. The wise saying *"knowledge is king"* definitely applied here, as I was gaining as much knowledge as I could about alternative treatments for my arthritic condition.

I remember very clearly one evening I was in my room contemplating the decision that I was up against. On one side of my bed was a stack of books on arthritis, and on the other side was a stack of books on natural approaches, including Dr. Gerson's book. It was like I had one of those balancing scales, and was weighing each side to see which would win. I think it was at this point I realized that the right thing for me to do was to try the natural approach. I could try it to see how my body would respond. It didn't feel like a big gamble for me, due to the fact that if the natural approach didn't work, I could always go back to taking medication. I also remember that night in my room re-reading one of the pamphlets the doctor gave me on arthritis titled *"Coping with Pain"*. It gave advice on how to cope with pain, and included information on how drugs help with the pain. I thought to myself, *"I don't want to take drugs and cope with the pain. I want to beat the pain, naturally!"* So that's what I set off to do.

The week had ended, and it was time for me to go back to the rheumatologist. I had only been on my medication for a month, which was minimal compared to some other patients I have read about. But even in that short time I was having issues with it. I was having stomach pains, trouble sleeping, and it made me nervous and jittery. At this point I noticed that my right toes and left pinky finger were starting to slightly deform, which really scared me. When I was doing my research, I had seen pictures in arthritis books of what some forms of incurable arthritis can do to the joints. It can deform the joints of the spine, hands and feet into obscure-looking structures that don't even resemble the originals. I definitely didn't want that to be my future, and I knew those unfortunate people had been on medications for years, and that's how they ended up. These pictures were a huge deciding factor in my decision to go with a natural program (I'm sorry to anyone out there whose hands or joints ended up like this. I feel that it is the medical establishment's wrong approach to disease that causes this to happen, and that's one of the reasons I am writing this book).

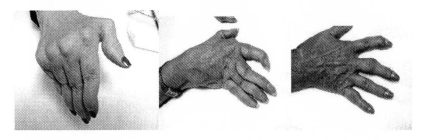

In 1996 the ACR (American College of Rheumatolgy) said that people who have active autoimmune arthritis marked by pain and swelling in multiple joints stand a greater than 70% chance of developing joint damage or bone erosions within two years of the beginning of the disease.

I was really looking forward to telling the rheumatologist what I had learned about this new natural program, and to see if he had ever heard of Dr. Max Gerson. I went into his office and waited for my appointment. They called my name, and I went into the exam room and waited for the doctor. He came in and began asking me questions to see how my body was feeling, and to make sure I was taking my medication. Then he performed some flexibility tests to determine the condition of my arthritis. Next, he asked me specifically about my medication to see if I had experienced any side effects or complications. I told him I was taking the medication twice a day, but I was having side effects and didn't like it. He said I could try a different type of medication to see how my body would react to it. At this point, things were about to get very complicated. I mentioned to him that I was talking to another type of doctor about a different type of program. I told him I went to a chiropractor that had a different way of dealing with arthritis. Immediately, the doctor's mood changed drastically. He crossed his arms and gave me an angry look, and said that a doctor of chiropractic is not a medical doctor, and doesn't have the proper training to give a diagnosis on arthritis. I wasn't even able to tell him about Dr. Max Gerson, and he already had a negative attitude. After the doctor hemmed and hawed about how he was expertly trained and that his way was the best way, I was finally able to mention Dr. Gerson and his natural approach. The doctor quickly stood up and said, "Natural way, that is quackery!" Then he said, "There is no proof or studies that document that the natural way works." I told him that it made sense to me, and at this point I had nothing to lose and wanted to give it a try anyway. Instantly the doctor rushed out of the room and left me sitting there alone. I sat there for at least twenty minutes, and then I started to get worried. I didn't know what was going on, so I got dressed and went out to the nurse to find out what happened. She told me that the doctor was finished with me, and she had me sign some papers and that was it. *I was stunned!* What ever happened to keeping an open mind to other programs? What ever happened to listening to a second opinion? I guess he was never taught that in medical school.

Looking back at this situation, I really owe that doctor a sincere thank you. What I mean by this is, if he hadn't left me just sitting there, and would have listened to me and tried to get me to continue taking medication on his program and maybe do a little bit of the natural program as well, then I probably wouldn't be writing this book today. I guess the doctor was upset because he thought he would be losing a lifelong patient, which I would have been if I had kept taking the medication (I will explain this further in the next chapter, on how taking medications is probably the biggest roadblock to letting the body heal itself naturally). Also, I really believe that when the doctor left me in the room by myself, it provided the fuel I needed to light a fire under me for the courage, desire, and motivation to choose a natural program. The medical establishment's traditional approach of medications and surgery didn't offer any promises or hope of a cure. I was not going to be a robot or a blind follower. The rheumatologist told me there was no cure, but I was going to find one. I guess it was time to *"not follow the doctor's orders!"*

4

Dr. Marcus Ettinger
The Gerson Program
Started

"I see in Dr. Max Gerson one of the most eminent geniuses in the history of medicine."
---Albert Schweitzer, M.D., Nobel Prize Laureate and former Gerson patient

To begin, I would like to reveal the name of the chiropractor that I have mentioned in the last few chapters. His name is Dr. Marcus Ettinger, and he's the one who opened my eyes to the natural approach and the Gerson program. This is a brilliant young chiropractor in Tustin, California, who had the courage and open-mindedness to believe in the power of natural healing. It's these types of people who are the real heroes in life.

It was now August of 1993. I was fired up and ready to start the natural program, but before I started I wanted to meet with Dr. Ettinger one more time. We sat down and went over the details of this new program. As I had already read and was familiar with Dr. Gerson's book from my first visit, it didn't take long for us to come up with a plan that I knew was realistic for me. It had to be a plan that I would be able to accomplish. If the plan was too difficult, then most likely I wouldn't adhere to it and would've just been wasting my time. The plan was now in place, and my mission had just begun.

Before I explain my journey into the natural world, I would like to briefly mention a few types of arthritis. I will not go into much detail, because most of the arthritis books out there, in which I'm sure some of you have already read, have complete chapters on the subject. The most common form is osteoarthritis. This is the kind that is known as the "wear and tear" type; the type you get from overuse and stress on your joints as you get older. Then there is seropositve polyarthritis (rheumatoid arthritis) and seronegative polyarthritis (without serum rheumatoid factors, the types that I was diagnosed with: ankylosing spondylitis and Reiter's syndrome). These types of arthritis are described as autoimmune forms, in which the body attacks itself and can leave your joints crippled or deformed, and can affect multiple organ systems. Reiter's syndrome can be self-limiting, frequently recurring, or develop continually. Repeated attacks over many years are common, and more than 40 percent of the patients end up with chronic and disabling arthritis, heart disease and impaired vision. *I now knew that the types of arthritis I had would eventually leave me a cripple, or seriously ill.* I also knew that time was of the essence, and that if I didn't act quickly that my joints would continue to deteriorate at a rapid pace. Up until now, it had only been about eight months since my first symptoms and I was already experiencing joint deformity in my toes and left pinkie. I was scared.

GERSON PROGRAM

This program was first developed over seventy years ago, and it is a shame that it is virtually unknown today. It was developed by Dr. Max Gerson, and used for cancer and other degenerative diseases such as arthritis, diabetes, multiple sclerosis, heart disease, etc. The idea of the program is to stimulate the body's own immune system to do what it usually does in a healthy body: *overcome disease.* By supplying the body with an overabundance of fresh vegetable juices, fruits, salads, organic foods and other supplements, the body will have the nutrients it needs to heal itself. Also, detoxification of the entire body is a crucial step of the program for the healing process to be effective. The program is not easy and requires full discipline, as it is a seven-day a week program. Remember, this program was first introduced for people who were extremely sick with cancer, so it is very intense.

This is what the Gerson program consists of:

- Vegetable Juices 13 Times Daily
- Organic Fruits and Vegetables
- Natural Foods Only
- Thyroid Tablets (ex: Armour Thyroid)
- Lugol's Iodine Solution
- Potassium Solution
- Vitamin B_{12}
- Crude Liver Extract
- Fresh Calf's Liver Juice
- Niacin
- Pancreatin Tablets (Digestive Enzymes)
- Lubile Capsules (Dried Powered Bile)
- Coffee Enemas
- No Medications

Note: Organic Iodine and Cholacol from Standard Process® may be substituted for Lugol's solution and Lubile capsules respectively. Armour Thyroid may only be prescribed by a physician.

I was not able to follow all of these items above at home, because that would have been unrealistic for me. I was not able to find fresh calf's liver juice, and juicing thirteen times per day was not an option. I'm not recommending that you deviate from the above program, because it is proven to work. What I am going to do is explain my version of the program. I highly suggest you read Dr. Gerson's book, *A Cancer Therapy: Results of Fifty Cases*, for the full details of the program.

My home version of the Gerson program consists of:

- Vegetable Juices 2 Times Daily, 64 oz. Total
- Organic Fruits and Vegetables
- Natural Foods Only
- Kelp Supplement
- Potassium Supplement
- Vitamin B-complex Supplement
- Crude Liver Extract Supplement
- Digestive Enzymes
- Coffee Enemas
- No Medications

Hippocrates stated, *"Let food be your medicine, and medicine be your food."* I knew at this point in my life that my lifestyle had to change completely to accommodate this theory and this new program. I was sick with arthritis, and didn't want to *just cope* with it the rest of my life. I was tired of dealing with the pain every day. Sometimes in life you have to get to the complete breaking point before you become motivated to change. I was at this breaking point, and I had to change my eating habits and stop eating all the unhealthy foods. No more junk food: pizza and beer, hamburgers, fries, and large cokes, fried foods, donuts, candy, alcohol, etc. This unhealthy food was all forbidden in this program and for good reason. In Dr. Gerson's words, "In the nutritional field, observations for centuries have shown that people who live according to natural methods in which plants, animals, and human beings are only fragments of the eternal cycle of nature, *do not get cancer*. On the contrary, people who accept methods of modern nutrition on an increasing scale become involved in degenerative diseases, including cancer, in a relatively short time."[1] And he further states, "Nutrition should be regarded as a remedy, prescribed as to kind and quantity or items to be forbidden."[2]

You may be wondering at this point, what foods are you supposed to eat on this program? That's a great question, and let me start by saying that the best way to approach this program is to look at the foods that *are* allowed. This will keep your mind positive and focused on your ultimate goal of becoming healthier. If instead you focus on the foods that are forbidden, then it will make the program harder to complete because you will always be thinking in the negative. We all know that in life you always want what you can't have, so let's not focus there (you can find the forbidden foods list on p. 238 of Dr. Gerson's book, or in this book. I give food choices in Chapter 10). Most of you know what foods are good and bad just by using common sense. This is a natural program, so you want to try to stay as close to nature as possible. No canned, processed, bottled, refined, or synthetic foods. Try to think of it like this: *if it comes out of a factory or has a long shelf life, then it isn't good for your body*. Here is a list of the main foods that I ate during the beginning of my program.

My home version of the Gerson foods consisted of:

- Vegetable Juices
- All Fruits and Vegetables
- Potatoes
- Oatmeal
- Wheat and Rye Bread
- Brown Rice and Wheat Pasta
- Nuts and Natural Peanut Butter
- Soy Milk
- Beans
- Eggs (organic)
- Chicken, Fish, and Turkey (not in the first few months and then only 1 or 2 times per week)
- Herbal Teas
- Honey for Sweetening

I began my program eating only these foods and cutting out anything unnecessary. In the words of Raquel Martin and Karen Romano, R.N., D.C., from their book, *Preventing and Reversing Arthritis Naturally*: "To survive, you need to become fit by raising your understanding above traditional medical dogma and going back to what is natural and pure for the body."[3] This is a hard concept to grasp. In a society that has been duped by the deceptive powers of the synthetic drug makers, it is hard to hear that *food is your best therapy*. All you have to do to follow this program is to stop eating meat and animal products, and start eating a large variety of uncooked, organically grown vegetables, fruits and sprouted nuts and seeds.[4] One of the reasons that you do not want to eat meat in the beginning of the program is because of a substance called *arachidonic acid*. Found almost exclusively in meats and most vegetable oils, arachidonic acid is a precursor to the "bad" kind of prostaglandins that produce platelet stickiness, hardening of the arteries, heart disease, and strokes, as well as inflammation.[5] So for me, I didn't eat any meat for the first few months. When I finally reintroduced meat back into my diet, I continued to not eat red meat or pork products, but instead ate chicken, fish, and turkey. I only ate meat one or two times per week, because meat is especially hard for people with arthritis to tolerate. In his book, *Optimum Health*, Stephen T. Sinatra says, "Although protein is important, arthritis and osteoporosis can develop if one eats too much acidic food such as meat and cheese; instead, eat alkaline foods such as barley grass, carrots, apple juice, and other fruits and vegetables."[6]

On another note, I would like to talk about sodium and potassium, and its importance in the body. Most of the products out there on the shelves today are loaded with sodium and lacking in potassium. *This sodium overload wreaks havoc on our bodies*. Dr. Gerson was very adamant and detailed about the balance of sodium versus potassium in the body. He says, "In a normal body all is alive, especially the basic substances built by the minerals, they have ionized or activated potassium and minerals of the potassium group with positive electrical potentials. In a sick body potassium is inactive – sodium and minerals of the sodium group are ionized with the possibilities of negative potentials.[7] The diet forms the basis of the medical treatment. It is based on the principal that sodium must be excluded as far as possible and the tissues must be enriched with potassium to the highest possible degree."[8] And in another statement about these minerals, Ralph Moss, Ph.D., states "Cells normally have a preference for potassium over sodium but when a cell is damaged it begins to prefer sodium."[9] My point is that you need to stick with natural foods, which are higher in potassium, and eliminate canned and processed foods, which are loaded with sodium.

At this point I had completely changed my eating habits and had focused on the nutritional part of the program. Now I needed to focus on another part of the program that was equally important, if not more, and definitely couldn't be overlooked. It is the detoxification process, and it is absolutely essential that both the nutritional and detoxification programs be done together if you wish to have any success at all. That was my next mission.

Detoxification Program

Let's say you have a slow leak in your car tire, and every morning you need to drive to the gas station to get it filled up so you can drive that day. Why would you do that? Wouldn't you just get the leak fixed? Yes, you would. That would be like fixing the symptom, which was the slow leak, and not fixing the problem, which was the hole in the tire. So I pose a question to everyone reading this, especially the doctors: Why would you just mask the symptoms of arthritis by giving patients medication every day? Wouldn't you rather fix the problem by improving their immune system, so that their bodies will get to the root of the problem and heal itself naturally? That's where detoxification fits into the equation.

Let's look at another analogy, this time between the human body and a car. The human body and a car are more similar than you might think: the body has a liver to filter the blood, and a car has an oil filter to clean the oil; the body has kidneys to filter the liquids it uses, and a car has a gas filter to clean its fuel; the body has lungs to filter the air it breathes, and a car has an air filter to clean the air it uses; the body has a stomach to mix the food it uses, and a car has a carburetor to mix the fuel it burns; the body has a colon to get rid of the wastes it excretes, and a car has an exhaust system to get rid of its wastes. What's my point? My point is that mechanics are trained and are smart enough to tell us that these filters need to be cleaned in order for that car to stay in top running condition. Then why don't doctors tell us to clean our body's filters to keep it running in top condition? Unfortunately, doctors are trained to just give us drugs that clog up our bodies even more. Again, that's where detoxification fits into the equation.

It was time for me to start the detoxification part of the program. In my situation, I was very fortunate that I was only on the medication for one month. I knew the Gerson program didn't allow medications to be taken, so I had to stop. This is when I learned a valuable lesson about how the immune system really works. As soon as I went off the medication, my body blew up with inflammation. My right foot looked like a bubble, and my left ankle was the size of a pineapple. They were both huge!

MY RIGHT TOES AND LEFT ANKLE

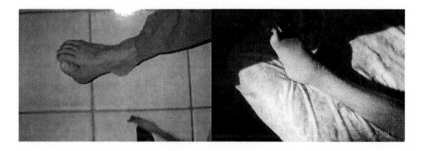

This is the results of taking medication! The medication that was prescribed to me was interfering with my body's natural inflammation process, so as soon as I stopped taking the medication, my body blew up to a shocking new level of inflammation. The reason was that since I was now off the medication, my body could function properly and knew that there was a problem in these areas. That's when it sent this extra swelling to protect the surrounding joints.

Most people might think that going off the medication is what caused my feet to swell up. Actually, it was just the opposite. Inflammation is natural, and it's our body's way of telling us that something is wrong. Inflammation is one of the ways the body protects itself after injury or disease.[10] It is the body's standard reactions to irritation. It basically consists of sending more blood to the area to flush away the irritants and to increase the supply of nutrients and white blood cells to speed healing. If the irritants are being produced faster than the blood can remove them, the inflammation can become chronic.[11] Since painkillers and anti-inflammatory medications are among the cornerstones of modern medicine, how can one even consider doing without them? Well, how about enabling the body's own immune system to work better, and how about stopping the cause of the inflammation alltogether?[12] Unfortunately, the painkillers and anti-inflammatory medications have problems. They temporarily relieve pain, but in the long run they simply cover up symptoms while the disease progresses further.[13] That was exactly what was happening in my body. The medication was holding back the inflammation that my body wanted to produce naturally. Permanent joint damage was occurring while I was on the medication, and I didn't even realize it because I couldn't feel the pain or see the inflammation. Let me say that again to re-emphasize it: *permanent joint damage was occurring while I was on the medication.*

Besides inflammation, let's talk about detoxification in further detail. Our bodies are extremely intelligent, and we need to listen to their signals to see what they are telling us. The body is always on guard to detoxify itself. Here are a few examples. When we eat something that is spoiled, or drink too much alcohol, the body will vomit to get rid of these toxins. When we have a bacteria or a virus in our stomach, or have overindulged in a particular food, the body will create diarrhea to get rid of the toxins. Fever and sweating are ways of getting rid of toxins, as heat will increase white blood cells, the immune system fighters. Coughing is trying to get the toxins we breathe out of the lungs.

And sneezing is getting rid of dust and irritants. So you see, the body is always trying to protect itself to survive.

In the beginning, the most important part of the program is an intensive detoxification of the entire body.[14] *Detoxification of the body refers to the cleansing of the bowels, kidneys, lungs, the liver, and the blood, since they are the organs involved in detoxification of chemicals and toxins from the body.* The liver acts as an "in-line" filter for the removal of foreign substances and wastes from the blood. The kidneys filter wastes from the blood into the urine, while the lungs remove volatile gases as we breathe.[15] Also, when detoxifying you will not feel as hungry. This is due to the fact that you are eating and drinking foods that have the proper nutrients, and not unhealthy food. As I mentioned before, the body is very smart, and it knows when it has the proper nutrients it needs to survive; and that's when it gives the signal to stop eating. The type of foods we avoid can also help the detoxification process. We should try to eliminate from our diets all sweets, like pie, cake, candy, ice cream, pastries, soft drinks, and sweet desserts of every variety. When it is possible, use honey on all foods you want to sweeten. It is both a sedative and a mild laxative, and promotes sound sleep at night.[16] Also, with the modern diet having excess animal proteins, fats, caffeine, alcohol, and chemicals, it inhibits the optimum function of our cells and tissues. The cleansing of toxins and waste products will restore our optimum function and vitality.[17]

One of the main causes of arthritis is an accumulation of toxic matter in various parts of the body. The only way to get permanent relief is to rid the body of these toxic wastes.[18] As Henry G. Bieler, M.D., states in his book, *Food is Your Best Medicine*, "As a practicing physician for over fifty years, I have reached three basic conclusions as to the cause and cure of disease. *The first is that the primary cause of disease is toxemia. My second conclusion is that in almost all cases the use of drugs in treating the patient is harmful.* Drugs often cause serious side effects, and sometimes even create new diseases. The dubious benefits they afford the patient are at best temporary. Yet the number of drugs on the market increases geometrically every year as each chemical firm develops its own variation of the compounds. *My third conclusion is that disease can be cured through the proper use of correct foods.* My conclusions are based on experimental and observational results, gathered through years of successfully treating patients."[19] I think we can assume that Dr. Bieler is in agreement with Dr. Gerson on the proper approach to stopping disease. So, the bottom line is that the only real way to true health is through internal cleansing and detoxification. All other methods are only temporary.[20]

I was now facing a major dilemma. My feet were so inflamed that I couldn't even walk. In fact, I couldn't even stand up on my own weight because they were so swollen and painful. Working was no longer an option, so I had to resign from the marketing job that I had been at the last couple of months. I remember trying to explain to my boss what I was going through. It didn't come out that well, and it kind of went like this, "Well, sir, I have to resign right now because I went off my medication and now I can't walk. I have arthritis and I am trying to defeat it the natural way. I have no idea how long it will take, and I hope I can continue employment there when I make it through my situation. Thanks for understanding." That was definitely a strange call I had to make, and it made me realize that our society doesn't have a clue as to what natural healing is all about. Well, I couldn't turn back now. It was crunch time, and I had to give the natural approach a 100% effort. You might be asking yourselves, how do I start this detoxification you're talking about? The answer is that is starts by cleaning the colon - and so that was my next mission.

Colon Program (Enemas)

Remember, in the movie "Beverly Hills Cop" with Eddie Murphy, the scene where he puts a banana in the car's tailpipe of the cops who were chasing him? Also, remember the exhaust pipe was so plugged up that when the cops tried to start the car, it caused the car to sputter and not start? It was a very funny scene. Our bodies work nearly the same as the car, but it's not funny in humans. If we have a plugged-up "tailpipe", so to speak, we will end up with all sorts of health problems. Think about all the unhealthy food that we eat in our society. This food does an excellent job of clogging up our colons and making them perform in a very sluggish fashion. This is the reason it is essential that we all clean them using this program.

Colon cleansing is an ancient and time-honored health practice for rejuvenating the system; it was used in Egypt over 4,000 years ago. Later, Hippocrates taught these procedures in his health care system. Using enemas, the large intestine, or colon, is healed, rebuilt, and finally restored to its natural size, normal shape, and correct function.[21] Enemas are found in world literature from Aristophanes to Shakespeare, Gulliver's Travels to Peyton Place.[22] Since you shower every day to clean the outside of your body, think of an enema as a shower for the inside of your body, but you don't do it as often. *A healthy colon is essential for the absorption of vital nutrients and the natural elimination of bodily waste and toxins.* Colon therapy promotes healthy colon function, and can ease a range of problems from headache and backache to arthritis and hypertension.[23] When the colon becomes burdened with an accumulation of waste material— impacted feces, bacteria, fungi, viruses, parasites, and dead cellular material—the result is termed "bowel toxemia." This condition causes inflammation and swelling of the bowel surface, and can lead to a host of other health problems.[24] "Colon therapy releases these toxins, cleanses the blood, stimulates the immune system, and aids in restoring the pH balance of the body", says Connie Allred, President of the American Colon Therapy Association. The colon is the sewer system of the body, and we all know how important it is to transport waste away.[25]

Keeping the bowels clean and moving is a major step in regaining our health, since the bowels are crucial in the elimination of toxins, especially those processed by the liver.[26] When we utilize colon therapy, the walls of the colon are washed, and old encrustations of fecal matter are loosened, dislodged, and swept away. This toxic waste material has often been attached to the bowel walls for many, many years. It is laden with millions of bacteria, which set up the perfect environment for disease to take root and entrench itself in the system, wreaking havoc. As the body pollution is eliminated, many conditions from severe skin disorders to breathing difficulties, depression, chronic fatigue, nervousness, severe constipation, and arthritis, are reduced in severity, providing great relief, especially when augmented with dietary changes and other treatment modalities.[27]

Since I was off medication, not even aspirin was allowed...but I was in a great deal of pain. Dr. Ettinger highly recommended *coffee enemas* to relieve the pain. I didn't have many options, so I made up my mind and just went for it. I clearly remember, one night, it was about two in the morning and I couldn't sleep because of the throbbing pain in my joints. I couldn't walk at this point in my program, so I had to crawl to the bathroom. I performed a coffee enema, and the pain was instantly relieved. I was amazed! *It worked better for pain relief than the medication I used to take.* Many of you out there might be shaking your heads, thinking that this is disgusting and that it's something you could never do. Keep in mind that I had a severe case of Reiter's Syndrome and Ankylosing Spondylitis, and my joints were deforming at a rapid pace. I didn't care or have time to contemplate whether it was disgusting. This was my life. I was going to do whatever it took to heal my body - and if that meant doing a couple of enemas a day for a month or so, then that was exactly what I was going to do.

After performing the coffee enemas, I had a new level of confidence in Dr. Ettinger, and also in Dr. Gerson. These doctors knew exactly what they were doing. In Dr. Gerson's own words, "Inasmuch as the detoxification of the body is of the greatest importance, especially in the beginning, it is absolutely necessary to administer frequent enemas, day and night (on the average, we give coffee enemas every four hours, day and night, and even more frequent against severe pain, nausea, general nervous tension and depression)."[28] The enema is a forgotten therapy that works wonders. Since the enema is generally held for 15 minutes, and all the blood passes through the liver every three minutes, these enemas represent a form of dialysis of blood across the gut wall.[29] There's little room left for doubt. A healthy colon is vital to living a life free of degenerative disease. If optimum health is your goal, then colon therapy could be most beneficial to you.[30]

Juicing Program

My next mission was to become an expert in the art of juicing. I'm sure many of you have seen this program advertised on television as "The Juice Man" type of products. I cannot stress enough the importance of juicing to obtain the nutrients needed to overcome disease. You might be thinking to yourselves that you eat plenty of vegetables, and this step of the program isn't necessary for you. I beg to differ. When you juice, it is in mass quantities. On average a person properly juicing using the Gerson program will consume on a weekly basis: 34 pounds of carrots, 25 pounds of apples, 1 head of red cabbage, 6 heads of lettuce, 1 bushel of celery, 1 bushel of parsley, and 2 pounds of green peppers, etc... You just can't eat that many vegetables in a week's time. *You have to juice them.*

Juicing works because the living nutrients in the fruits and vegetables get into the bloodstream and down to the cellular level immediately. The body does not have to expend energy or time to process food through the whole digestive system.[31] Juiced produce contains hundreds of vitamins, minerals, and phytochemicals that are essential for maintaining a healthy body. These chemicals are vital to healthy organs and cells, as well as to a strong immune system.[32] Juice therapy can be very helpful with congestion of colds and flus, recurrent infections, allergies, skin disorders, and gastrointestinal problems, as well as other congestive or chronic disorders.[33]

The goal of the Gerson program is to juice thirteen times a day. Unfortunately, I was only able to juice twice a day. But when I juiced it was thirty-two ounces, so I was consuming a total of sixty-four ounces of fresh juices daily. It's important to buy the correct kind of juicer as well. The Gerson program recommends a separate grinder and press to prepare the juices. That's the best kind, because it sustains the most enzymes and nutrients, and I recommend that you try to use this type of juicer when you start the program. With the resources that I had available at the time, I was only able to purchase the centrifugal type of juicer. These are the popular type of juicers on the market and are otherwise know as "The Juice Man" type. This type worked well for me, even though the benefits might not be as great compared to the press-type juicers. Regardless, the goal is to juice and to do it daily. Below I have listed my top five reasons for juicing.

My Top 5 Benefits of Juicing

1. **Nutritional Powerhouse**
   The rich juices contain high concentrations of vitamins, minerals, trace elements, and enzymes that help detoxify and heal the body.

2. **Easy Assimilation**
   Since the juice is in liquid form, it takes little or no time for these nutrients to enter the bloodstream and be utilized by the body. Since digestion takes an abundant amount of energy, drinking these juices will free your body of this digestion time and give you greater energy.

3. **Live Enzymes**
   Live enzymes are found abundantly in fresh fruits and vegetables. These enzymes are used to help digest and clean the system. Enzymes are the "spark plugs" of life that give us the energy to keep moving.

4. **Total Detoxification**
   Due to the live enzymes and abundant nutrients in the juices, inner cleansing will be much quicker and your overall detoxification program will be more effective.

5. **Lose Weight**
   When you drink fresh juices on a daily basis you are getting the proper nutrients that the body needs. Once your body receives these nutrients it will be satisfied and will not feel hungry. This is one of the easiest ways to lose weight.

SAUNA PROGRAM (Hyperthermia)

I was now only a few weeks into my program of eating natural foods, juicing, and colon cleansing. My treatment was going extremely well. I learned from Dr. Gerson's book that the healing process was not a quick one. *Healing the body can take up to a year to a year and a half, and is a lifelong program.* You can't just do the program and then go right back to your poor eating and lifestyle choices, and hope that everything will be fine. You have to make a commitment to better health and stick with it.

I wasn't working at this time, and my only focus was doing the programs and trying to heal my body. I had another appointment with Dr. Ettinger, and it was another one I will never forget. I was still unable to walk due to the inflammation in my right foot and left ankle, so when I arrived at Dr. Ettinger's office it was quite unusual. He pushed an office chair with wheels out to my car, since I didn't have access to a wheelchair. In fact, I didn't want access to a wheelchair in the fear of mentally surrendering to arthritis, so the office chair with wheels was my only option (it wasn't likely that someone was going to carry me into the office, being that I was 6'6" and weighed 215 pounds). I was pushed into his office, and Dr. Ettinger explained the next step of the program to me in more detail. It was called the Hubbard Purification Program, and Dr. Ettinger had just completed the program himself. *I love a doctor who practices what he preaches!*

This was not part of the Gerson program; this was taught to me exclusively by Dr. Ettinger. The program consisted of a few steps. First, you would take varying levels of niacin (vitamin B_3), which induces a flush to the skin, opening up the capillaries and mobilizing toxins. Then you would exercise from twenty to thirty minutes to get the blood flowing. Next you would sit in a dry heat sauna for up to three hours per day. During the three hours you would alternate between sitting in the sauna for twenty to thirty minutes and then exiting and taking a cool shower for five minutes. The cool shower allows your body temperature to come back down to normal. Finally, you would rest for a few minutes outside of the sauna. This was the procedure, and you would repeat this five times per session. It was very important to drink plenty of water during the session, because you would have a high level of perspiration. The whole concept is to mobilize and sweat out accumulated residues of past drugs, medicines, alcohol, and radiation.

So I called the facility that Dr. Ettinger recommended, and signed up for the program. My first visit to the sauna program was also a visit I wouldn't forget. Once again, I was still unable to walk so they had to push an office chair with wheels out to the curb, just like Dr. Ettinger. They had to push me into the clinic. It was a very humbling experience, and taught me how fortunate I was to be able to walk before this arthritis. It was quite a change for me, considering I was running up and down the basketball court just nine months earlier.

Sauna therapy is great for removing toxins from the skin and regenerating one's health and energy. With that in mind, it is important to know that the skin is the biggest organ of the body and is made up of over four million pores that are constantly acting as the cooling system for the body.[34] It has been documented that our skin's sweat glands, when combined, can perform as much detoxification as one (or both) kidneys.[35] The body's sweat glands are an important part of the cleansing system. Most people associate the kidneys with elimination of toxic waste. By using the body's sweat glands, it is possible to cleanse the body even better.[36] So, sauna therapy is an excellent way to stimulate the release of toxins from the cells and allow their elimination, first through the skin, and later through the bowels and kidneys.[37]

Release of impurities is just one of the things that sweat therapy accomplishes. The artificial "fever" that sauna bathing induces appears to have immune-system stimulating properties similar to those of a "natural" fever. There is growing recognition of the role fever plays in the process of healing. During a fever, production of white blood cells increases, along with the rate of their release into the bloodstream. The disease-fighting capacity of white blood cells increases, and the body's production of interferon and antibodies also speeds up.[38] The great physician Paramenides, 2,000 years ago, said, "Give me a chance to create a fever and I will cure any disease." High temperature speeds up metabolism and inhibits the growth of an invading virus and bacteria. *Such giants of medical science as Nobel Prize winner Dr. A. Lwoff, Dr. Werner Zabel, and Dr. Josef Issels, recommend and use fever therapies extensively.*[39]

Regular saunas may also improve blood flow to the heart and prevent heart disease, according to Japanese researchers. "The benefits of repeated sauna therapy are similar to those of exercise," says Dr. Chuwa Tei of Kagoshima University in Japan. But saunas have an advantage because they can be used to treat people who have trouble walking, and they do not overload the heart.[40] I definitely fit into the category of not being able to walk, so this program was a perfect match for me. According to a study published in *The Journal of American College of Cardiology*, men with risk factors for coronary heart disease may improve circulation by taking regular saunas.[41] So the sauna program isn't just for releasing toxins; it also helps improve circulation and preventing heart disease. And just think, all of these benefits for just sitting around relaxing in a dry heat sauna.

This Hubbard Purification Program took me two months to complete. It was a long two months, due to the fact that it was a seven-day a week program at three hours per day. During the program, I noticed many health benefits occurring. Each week I could tell that my health was improving: my skin looked healthier, my eyes became clearer, I had more energy, the arthritis pain was diminishing, and of course the inflammation and swelling decreased. As I was sitting in the sauna three hours each night, I could almost feel the toxins rushing out through my pores. It was very refreshing. It took just two weeks on this sauna program (of course I was still following the Gerson protocol) before the swelling went down in my feet to the point where I was able to walk on my own again. So in retrospect, I was unable to walk for a period of a month and a half. I sure was excited that chapter of my life was over.

5

Dr. Lis Baird
Kinesiology and Herbology
Explored

"The physician is only nature's assistant."
---Galen, legendary physician 131-201 A.D.

It was now November of 1993. I had been on my natural program for three months, and I was excited because I knew deep down that the worst was behind me. I knew that the program was working effectively, and the pain medication was no longer needed. It's hard to describe the feeling you get when you know that you have found a program that is healing your body daily. *All without the use of harmful drugs*! My future was looking brighter every day. One thing that you might be wondering is: after eating natural foods for three months, was I craving for the foods I used to eat like fast foods, sodas, candy, alcohol, etc? To a small degree, yes I was. But, did I let my taste buds take over and indulge in these foods? No, because I knew that if I had eaten these types of foods again, that it would only hurt my chances for recovery. I had to be disciplined and have the mindset that if I ate these unhealthy foods, I would be going backwards in my healing program. I sure didn't want to go backwards to the point of not being able to walk again. I looked at my situation as day-to-day decisions to either eat healthy foods to help my body heal or eat unhealthy foods and continue to suffer with arthritis. The decision to eat the healthy foods was unanimous.

I was fortunate to be working again. I had contacted my old manager at the marketing company and explained to him that my arthritis had greatly improved due to the natural programs that I had been undergoing. He was a little confused as to how natural programs could help with an incurable disease, but he was happy that I was doing better. Life was moving forward once again. I settled into a routine of going to work, doing my natural programs, and slowly healing day-by-day. One weekend I met my best friend, Brad, at a coffee shop to talk and catch up on old times. I was so focused on my programs that I hadn't had much time for him or any other of my friends over the last few months. He knew what I was going through, and that I was treating my arthritis with only natural programs. This was about the time my future was about to get brighter once again. Brad mentioned that he knew a doctor who specialized in natural programs and had helped him with a back problem about a year earlier. He thought she would be a perfect fit into my overall plan. I agreed, and gave her a call to set up an appointment at the earliest available date.

The name of Brad's friend was Dr. Lis Baird, and she was a doctor of chiropractic who specialized in kinesiology, herbology, and nutrition. I headed off to my appointment knowing I had at least a forty-five minute drive that awaited me. I drove a stick shift car at the time, and with my left ankle still a bit painful, the shifting wasn't much fun. I'm glad there wasn't much traffic on the freeway that day; otherwise my ankle would have been throbbing by the time I arrived. I made it to her office, sat down, and waited for my appointment. I still had a slight limp when I walked. When I met with her, the first thing I noticed was her amazing energy level and great big smile. You could tell that this was someone who really enjoyed her work. Before I even had a chance to explain my situation, she asked me if I had some kind of arthritis. My friend Brad never told her about my arthritis, so I was amazed that she could recognize my condition so quickly. I guess she must have noticed it when I first came into her office. This is truly astonishing to me, that Dr. Baird took the time and paid special attention to me, especially considering I had never seen or met her before, and I wasn't even a patient of hers yet. I know many traditional doctors out there today are so overwhelmed with patients that they only have a few minutes for each one. Patients today are almost viewed as a number. Well, that was not the case with Dr. Baird.

So I told her that I did indeed have arthritis, and further explained my entire experience the last year of my life. I explained how I was working with another doctor of chiropractic, and how he introduced me to the Gerson program. I asked her if she had ever heard of Dr. Max Gerson, and she quickly turned to her book shelf and pulled out his book. She explained that it was an incredible program and that I should, by all means, continue using it. This was awesome! *It was the biggest relief to me that another doctor had not only heard of Dr. Gerson, but also highly recommended it.* Remember, most people I had told about my program so far had no idea what I was experiencing, and even thought I was crazy for going against traditional medicine. I was confident that Dr. Baird would fit into my program perfectly. My next mission was to learn the programs that she had to offer in my pursuit to defeat my arthritis.

BENEFITS OF CHIROPRACTIC

Since both Dr. Ettinger and Dr. Baird are amazing doctors of chiropractic that helped me experience new levels of health, I would like to briefly explain the benefits of chiropractic care. The greatest benefits of chiropractic care occur when used as a preventive tool. The spine's primary function is to protect the spinal cord and nerve roots. Because chiropractic adjustments improve spinal alignment and function, they can also reduce stress and irritation of the spinal nerve roots, thereby promoting overall health and wellness.

When there is no nerve interference, your nervous system controls the healthy function of virtually every cell, tissue, organ, and system of your body. Therefore, any problem can be improved with a better functioning nervous system. Chiropractic helps the nervous system function better by removing blockages that may be preventing you from good health.

Some of the main benefits of chiropractic:

- Postural Correction
- Greater Flexibility
- Freedom of Movement
- Stress Reduction
- Improved Sleep
- Enhanced Immune System
- Increased Energy
- Relief from Headaches
- Recovery from Trauma

I feel that quite often, doctors of chiropractic get overlooked or frowned upon by the medical establishment. This might be because many chiropractors refrain from using drugs, but instead use natural healing methods. Regardless of the reason, it's an absolute shame because there is no drug available that doctors can prescribe that will help the nervous system in the long run better than chiropractic adjustments. Besides, chiropractic adjustments don't have the harsh side effects that drugs do, which only strengthens the appeal of this program.

APPLIED KINESIOLOGY

Dr. Baird revealed her first program to me, and it was called applied kinesiology. This technique was first developed by George Goodheart, D.C., in 1964, and is the study of the relationship between muscle dysfunction (weak muscles) and related organ or gland dysfunction. It employs a simple strength resistance test on a specific indicator muscle related to the organ or part of the body that is being tested.[1] It can determine health imbalances in the body's organs and glands by identifying weakness in the specific muscles. By stimulating or relaxing these key muscles, an applied kinesiologist can recognize and resolve a variety of health problems.[2] The muscle-gland-organ link can indicate the cause of the health problem and lead to further diagnostic tests for confirmation. Once the problem is identified, it can be treated by a variety of techniques to strengthen the muscles involved and restore health.[3] *Applied kinesiology does not cure any disease. Rather, it provides a way for the doctor to evaluate and restore proper function of the nervous system, thereby allowing the body to once again regulate its own health.*

Some of the main benefits of kinesiology:

- Improve Posture and Range of Motion
- Restore Normal Function of the Nervous, Immune, and Digestive Systems
- Determine Unsuspected Food Sensitivities
- Enhance Blood Circulation
- Relieve Muscle Spasms
- Correct Chronic Pain
- Improve Meridian Energy Flow

This was another program that I had to view with an open mind. All these natural programs were new to me, and each one was another piece of the puzzle to defeat my arthritis. When Dr. Baird performed the kinesiology examination, I was a little apprehensive at first. She would have me hold my arm straight out, push down on it while she tested my different organ and gland systems, and then determine if everything was working properly. If there were any imbalances, she would use her chiropractic skills to correct them. The test seemed too simple to do anything for me. But after several visits and corrections to my body, I realized that it was very effective. The slight pain that I did have seemed to diminish, and my energy level was greater than it had been in months. I was extremely happy with my results thus far, and my next mission was to see what other programs Dr. Baird had in store for me.

HERBOLOGY

Dr. Baird's next program was herbology. It is the world's oldest system of medicine, and has been in use for more than 5,000 years. In the 1940s, herbology lost its medical prominence in the U.S. with the advent of antibiotics. However, modern researchers are finding that herbology is safer, less expensive and at minimum as effective as prescription drugs. Today, approximately 25 percent of all prescription drugs are still derived from trees, shrubs, or herbs.[4] This percentage shows you how effective herbs can be, and should never be overlooked.

A major aspect of the philosophy of herbology is the treatment of the person as a whole, rather than treating only the symptoms. The herbalist seeks to treat the underlying cause of disease or ill health. Remember my analogy from the last chapter regarding the tire, and fixing the problem and not the symptom. Herbology directly applies to this analogy. Fundamental to herbology is the belief that the body has an innate ability to heal itself; therefore, treatment should enhance this quality. When treating chronic illness with herbology, it is extremely important to treat the entire body, as the illness may be simultaneously affecting many systems of the body at various levels.[5] "Because herbs and plants use an indirect route to the bloodstream and target organs, their effects are usually slower in onset and less dramatic than those of purified drugs administered by more direct routes. Doctors and patients accustomed to the rapid, intense effects of synthetic medicines may become impatient with botanicals for this reason."[6]

I already had a basic understanding of herbology from the research I had previously done, but Dr. Baird further expanded my knowledge. She was an enthusiast in herbology, and was able to determine which herbs my body actually needed for better health. She accomplished this by combining her applied kinesiology skills and herbal knowledge together, as one force. It was amazing to see her use these skills together. I certainly like programs like these in which the results are right in front of your own eyes. The body doesn't lie, and it responds to what it needs to become stronger and improve its health. Dr. Baird has dedicated her life to becoming an expert in these specialties so she can improve the quality of life for others. That is the reason she is such a special person to me. All I can say is that I was extremely lucky to have Dr. Baird on my health team to help defeat my arthritis.

Specific Arthritis Herbs

There are hundreds of herbs available for you to use in your quest for better health. In fact, there are many books in which the subject is entirely devoted to herbs and herbology. I recommend that you read those types of books if you are looking for more details. In this next section, I am only going to mention the herbs that I used throughout my program. I didn't take all of these herbs at the same time, so don't worry about having to take handfuls of pills everyday. I would mix and match and try different combinations to see which ones worked best for me. *Healing the body and maintaining good health is a life-long process.* The key is that these herbs are all very effective at improving and maintaining good health, and should be utilized by anyone who is serious about their own health.

Alfalfa

Alfalfa is also known as the "great healer". It is one of the most mineral-rich foods known to man, due to the fact that its roots grow as deep as 130 feet into the earth. It contains calcium, magnesium, phosphorus, and potassium, plus all known vitamins. The minerals are in a balanced form, which promotes better absorption. It has helped many arthritis sufferers.[7] According to a recent study that appeared in the scientific journal *Atherosclerosis,* not only is alfalfa rich in minerals, but it's also a potent natural cholesterol buster. Researchers gave 15 patients with high cholesterol 40 grams of alfalfa seeds three times daily for eight weeks.

The result: the median total cholesterol declined by 17 percent; and better yet, the LDL or bad cholesterol dropped by 18 percent.[8]

Cayenne

This is also known as the "hottest healer". It can be used as a supplement or in topical form to treat areas of pain. "Cayenne has proved so effective at relieving pain that it's the active ingredient in the over-the-counter cream Zostrix," says James A. Duke, Ph.D., a retired botanist from the U.S. Department of Agriculture and author of *The CRC Handbook of Medicinal Herbs.*[9] Also, cayenne may help the heart. "It cuts cholesterol levels and reduces the risk of internal blood clots that trigger heart attack," says Daniel B. Mowrey, PhD., director of the American Phytotherapy Research Laboratory in Salt Lake City, and author of *The Scientific Validation of Herbal Medicine.*[10]

I have heard many people say that they don't want to take cayenne because they feel it may upset their stomachs. This is a rumor that is entirely not true. In fact, it's just the opposite with cayenne, as it is very beneficial for stomach disorders. Varro E. Tyler, Ph.D., professor of pharmacognosy at Purdue University School of Pharmacy and author of *The Honest Herbal*, believes cayenne to be a stomach-settling digestive aid. He states, "It stimulates the flow of saliva and stomach secretions. Saliva contains enzymes that begin the breakdown of carbohydrates, and stomach secretions contain acids and other digestive substances."[11] And to elaborate further, UCLA researcher Dr. Irving Ziment recommends using cayenne (chilis) to help alleviate the symptoms of a common cold. Dr. Ziment says, "Chilies can help break up congestion and keep the airways clear."[12]

Devil's Claw

This amazing herb is also known as the "grapple plant." Devil's claw is approved as a nonprescription medicine by the German

Commission E, which is an expert panel of physicians and pharmacists. The German Commission E also advises the U.S. Food and Drug Administration. Approved uses of devil's claw include loss of appetite, digestive disorders, and degenerative disorders that include pain and inflammation in the joints.[13] *Many arthritis patients show a remarkable decrease in joint swelling when they use devil's claw.*[14]

According to Mark Blumenthal, founder and executive director of the American Botanical Council, a nonprofit research and education organization, "At least two previous clinical trials on devil's claw have supported its use as an aid in treating lower back pain and rheumatic conditions." The clinical study was published in an issue of *Phytomedicine*, a leading European journal dealing with scientific research on herbs and phytomedicinal products.[15] Another clinical study adds to the growing body of evidence supporting the use of devil's claw root in osteoarthritis. The double blind, randomized trial concluded that devil's claw was as effective in relieving pain, and safer than diacerhein (a type of drug known as a symptomatic slow-acting drug for osteoarthritis, or SYSADOA). Results showed that the two treatments were equally effective in relieving spontaneous pain. However, by the end of the study, significantly fewer people in the devil's claw group needed to take additional analgesics for "rescue" pain relief.[16]

Feverfew

Feverfew is known in the herbal world as the "headache herb." In an interesting study done in 1984 at the City of London Migraine Clinic, researchers used patients who had already achieved relief from headaches by taking feverfew and gave them either feverfew or a placebo. Researchers tracked the patient's progress for several months. What was the final result? Migraine patients taking the placebo saw their migraine headaches return.[17]

But it's not just for headaches. Researchers in the United Kingdom have identified a new flavonol in the plant called tanetin, which contributes to the anti-inflammatory action of feverfew. In the U.K., feverfew is also used by consumers for the treatment of arthritis because of perceived anti-inflammatory effects. This study, published in the January 1995 issue of *Phytochemistry*, provides evidence for the presence of a compound in the plant to which anti-inflammatory activity can be attributed.[18] Feverfew is also found to be beneficial in relieving menstrual cramps, preventing blood clots, rheumatic disease, and allergies.[19] This is just another example of how an herbal supplement can add to your arsenal of weapons in your fight against disease.

Garlic

This herb, without a doubt, is the undisputed champion at fighting disease and improving our immune systems. It is also known as the "king of herbs." Garlic contains many sulfur compounds, which give it its marvelous healing properties. *This herb is good for virtually any and all diseases and infections. It is so common in Russia that it is known as "Russian penicillin".*[20] Studies confirm the immune stimulation provided by garlic. Subjects receiving aged garlic extract at 1800 mg a day for three weeks showed a 155.5% increase in natural killer immune cell activity that kills invaders and cancer cells.[21]

Garlic contains a wide range of substances, including antioxidants, that act together to help prevent arteriosclerosis, heart disease, stroke, cancer and aging, as well as boost immunity and help increase memory and life span.[22] "When you feel a sore throat coming on, eat some garlic to scare off your cold or flu. If you do it early enough, you may not even get sick," says James North, chief of microbiology at Brigham Young University in Provo, Utah. For example, Dr. North found that garlic extract kills nearly 100% of both a human rhinovirus, which causes colds, and Para influenza-3, a flu and respiratory virus.[23]

In our world today, I feel that most doctors over-prescribe antibiotics. I feel that these doctors are stuck in the habit of writing out prescriptions without using all the available options to them. But of course, doctors are trained to prescribe drugs, so this isn't a big surprise. *Doctors get paid if they write out a prescrip-*

tion, and get nothing for recommending a natural product like garlic. Antibiotics kill off the good bacteria as well as the bad, and allow the bad to repopulate and develop antibiotic resistance. Natural forms of antibiotics are better, since they do not kill off the good bacteria with the bad and do not allow drug resistance to take place. Garlic, for example, is perhaps 200 times more effective against bacteria and virus than most antibiotics today.[24]

Another incredible benefit of garlic is its effects on the heart. Benjamin Lau, M.D., professor at California's Loma Linda University School of Medicine, where he taught medical microbiology and immunology, tells us, "With the use of garlic, preferably on a daily basis, you will promote scrubbing action that will help control the levels of cholesterol sludge to protect against cardiovascular distress."[25] Further, "Clinical studies are in agreement that there's something in garlic that helps prevent blood clotting," says Eric Block, Ph.D., State University of New York at Albany.[26]

Garlic is so essential to good health that everyone should consume it, even though it has a strong odor. There are garlic supplements on the market that are odorless, so you do have options. Let's assume for some strange reason that I was left stranded on a tropical island and I had no other forms of medication. All I had were the clothes on my back, and I had to learn to live off the land to survive. If I became ill, I would be in serious trouble. If I only had one item to choose from for my future medications, without a doubt I would choose garlic. It works effectively as a natural antibiotic, and is diverse enough to heal many conditions of the body. It's just that good!

Ginger

This herb is known as the "universal medicine herb." This is true, because the benefits of ginger are numerous. Some of the benefits include: ease nausea, calm the stomach, promote the flow of bile, improve the appetite, help support a healthy cardiovascular system and improve circulation, help inflammatory joint diseases such as arthritis, and lower blood cholesterol.

Ginger mends joints, inhibits pain-producing prostaglandins, and works as an anti-inflammatory. *Clinical studies report that patients have received more relief from pain, swelling, and stiffness from taking ginger than from synthetic NSAIDs.*[27] It also has properties of aspirin but without the side effects. A researcher at Cornell University Medical College discovered that ginger has an effect on blood clots that is similar to that of aspirin.[28] In another study, Dr. Krishna C. Srivastava of Odense University in Denmark, an internationally known medical researcher on spices, says, "Try ginger to relieve your rheumatoid arthritis. It's an anti-inflammatory agent."[29]

A Danish study found that ginger ingestion is significant in relieving pain associated with rheumatoid arthritis, osteoarthritis and muscular disorder patients. In this study, 56 patients (28 rheumatoid, 18 osteo, 10 muscular) were studied over periods ranging from 3 months to 2.5 years. Three-quarters of the 56 arthritis patients experienced relief in pain and swelling. All of the muscular discomfort patients experienced relief in pain. Over the period of the testing, no patients reported any adverse effects from consistent ginger consumption.[30]

Milk Thistle Extract

Milk thistle is also known as "nature's liver protector." A leading expert on health and nutrition, Gary Null, said in *Spectrum* magazine: "Milk thistle heals the liver in three ways. First, it stabilizes and strengthens the membranes of liver cells, preventing the entry of damaging toxins. Second, milk thistle is a powerful antioxidant that neutralizes free radicals. It is many times more powerful than vitamin E in this respect. Third, milk thistle speeds the regeneration of damaged liver tissue by initiating cellular protein synthesis."[31] This is a powerful statement, considering the liver's vital importance to the body. The liver is the human body's great detoxifier. All foods, liquids, oral drugs, pollutants and pesticides pass through the liver as they travel from the intestines into the bloodstream. Blood passes through the liver at a rate of about three pints per minute. At any instant, the liver contains about ten percent of all the blood in the human body.[32] A poorly functioning liver usually equates to poor health.

Scandinavian researchers tested milk thistle extract's effect on livers that were stressed but not seriously diseased. They selected 106 consecutive patients who had abnormal liver-function tests from alcohol use, but who did not have cirrhosis. Half took milk thistle extract; the other half received a placebo. After four weeks, the placebo group showed no change in liver function, but the milk thistle group showed highly significant improvement, and in some cases complete normalization of liver function, despite their alcohol consumption.[33] A 1989 report in the *Journal of Hepatology* described a study involving 170 people with advanced alcoholic cirrhosis, an often fatal condition. The study participants were divided into two groups. One received 200 mg of milk thistle extract three times a day, the other received a medically inactive look-alike placebo. Both groups were followed for four years. During that time, the death rate in the placebo group was about 60 percent, but among those taking the milk thistle extract, only 40 percent died, a highly statistically significant difference.[34] A 20 percent improvement rate might not seem too significant, but don't forget this was with patients that had advanced alcoholic cirrhosis, not normal livers.

"Milk thistle extract is a powerful antioxidant," says Alan R. Gaby, M.D., a Baltimore physician who practices nutritional and natural medicine and is president of the American Holistic Medical Association. "Antioxidants counter the effects of naturally occurring toxins called free radicals. In animal studies, it has prevented liver damage, and in human studies, it has sped recovery from hepatitis," says Dr. Gaby.[35] Laboratory studies by Bharat B. Aggarwal, Ph.D., a professor of cancer medicine at the University of Texas M.D. Anderson Cancer Center in Houston, and his colleagues suggest that milk thistle extract acts on biochemical pathways to aid in detoxification. In the laboratory, milk thistle extract is quite protective against liver damage. It is approved in Europe by The German Commission E for liver damage - especially that induced by alcohol - and seems to have no adverse effects.[36]

White Willow Bark

This is an interesting herb, also known as "nature's aspirin." It has been given this name because it contains acetyl-salicylic acid, the active ingredient in aspirin.[37] *It has been used in China for centuries as a medicine because of its ability to relieve pain and lower fever.* The salicylic acid in white willow bark lowers the body's levels of prostaglandins, hormone-like compounds that can cause aches, pain, and inflammation. While white willow bark takes longer to begin acting than aspirin, its effect may last longer. And, unlike aspirin, it doesn't cause stomach bleeding or other known adverse effects.[38] Many arthritis sufferers taking white willow bark have experienced reduced swelling and in-flammation, and eventually increased mobility.

Experts point out that white willow bark will work on al-most anything or any condition in which you have used aspirin. What I don't understand is if it works as well as aspirin without the side effects, then why was aspirin ever invented? Why is eve-ryone haphazardly taking it for aches and pains? *Did you know that 46 people die every day from aspirin alone in the USA?[39]* And if that's not terrible enough, used over long periods of time, aspirin may depress the production rate of immune bodies of the immune system, thus undermining the body's own healing pow-ers. By masking symptoms of the acute stages of arthritis, it leads the patient to a false sense of security and actually contributes to conversion of the disease to a chronic stage.[40] The pharmacies and drug stores should all be stocked with bottles of white willow bark supplements, not aspirin. Why does mankind always have to fool with nature? Sometimes things are better left untouched, and this would be one of them.

James A. Duke, Ph.D., a botanist retired from the U.S. Department of Agriculture and author of *The CRC Handbook of Medicinal Herbs*, states: "I have used willow bark for toothache pain, and if I were at risk, I would drink willow bark tea for heart attack prevention."[41] There are more reasons than ever to use this herb. Medical research shows that the chemical in white willow not only reduces fever and relieves pain and inflammation, but also may help prevent heart attack, stroke, digestive tract cancers and migraine headaches. The benefits of taking white willow far exceed that of aspirin. So the next time you reach for your aspirin bottle, think twice about it and instead try using the natural supplement.

Yucca

This herb is known as the "blood purifying herb" and is routinely prescribed for arthritis in health clinics. The powerful intestinal cleansing effect of yucca can eliminate the toxins built up in our digestive tract. The cleansing effect in turn reduces the toxins that our body absorbs into our blood stream through our intestinal walls. *The result is an effective detoxification, which is the beginning of all healing processes.*

John W. Yale, Ph.D., a botanist in Porterville, California, made a special study and found that yucca contained a high potency of naturally occurring plant saponin. The anti-stress property of this plant saponin may account for yucca's health and medical applications.[42] Clinical research resulted in evidence that the saponin in yucca could not only reduce stress and swelling of joints in people, but could also lower the tendency to develop toxic wastes in the colon. At the National Arthritis Medical Clinic in Desert Hot Springs, California, Robert Bingham, M.D., and Bernard A. Bellew, M.D., leading yucca researchers, devised tests to determine if yucca could be of benefit in the treatment of arthritis. According to their report published in the *Journal of Applied Nutrition*, 60 percent of the people who took the yucca supplement experienced diminished pain, swelling, and stiffness. There were no side effects. Furthermore, those who took the yucca extract supplement had lower blood pressure and cholesterol levels, and relief from intestinal toxicity.[43]

6

Gary Richer
The Live Cell King

"The real units of life consist of millions of small entities in the visible cells."
---Thomas Edison, 1,093 U.S. patents,
more than any other person

I t was now February of 1994. I was six months into this natural program and my progress was going incredible well. I was still fully utilizing the Gerson programs that Dr. Ettinger taught me, including juicing, detoxification, and the natural foods. In addition, using Dr. Baird's kinesiology over the past three months, we were able to determine my body's weaknesses, fine-tune them, and strengthen them to the highest possible level. Also, I incorporated the herbology that she introduced to me and was taking herbs on a daily basis as well. Given my current condition based on pain and swelling, using a scale of 1 to 10, I would say that I was about a 6. It sure was nice not having to crawl around the house on my hands and knees like I did the first month and half. So I looked into the future and assumed that it would probably take another six months of this program before I was 100 percent. That's an improvement rate of about 8-10 percent a month. That might seem slow to some of you, but keep in mind that the healing process takes time and doesn't happen overnight. *There are no "magic bullets" to take that will heal you immediately.* In these six months, I had a few ups and downs. I would go through episodes known as "healing crisis" periods. These were periods when the body was in an extreme healing mode. It would cause more pain than normal and be accompanied by other symptoms, such as feeling weak and having flu-like symptoms. They would usually only last a couple of days and then afterwards my body would be much stronger. You have to understand that healing crisis periods are normal and are signals from your body that it's detoxifying and healing itself. It definitely wasn't fun to go through these periods, but I knew deep down in my heart that it would be all right, because I was providing my body with the nutrients and programs it needed to overcome my arthritis.

As I was completing my programs with Dr. Baird, she knew that I still had a struggle in front of me. She also knew that I was open to new ideas and any natural program that would help improve my health condition. At that point, my life was about to change for the better once again. She had a friend who was an expert in his line of work and she thought his programs might be a benefit to me. One of the programs utilized a microscope to see the quality of your blood, and the other program was a technique on finding genetic weaknesses and strengthening them. I was excited about getting the chance to meet this expert and to learn his natural programs. I jumped at the opportunity and called him to set up an appointment. My journey continued into the natural world of health.

LIVE CELL ANALYSIS

As I walked into his office, I immediately had a gut feeling that I just gained another team member in my quest for better health. His name was Gary Richer and his smile was very friendly, just like Dr. Ettinger and Dr. Baird. What was it with these natural doctors always smiling? I guess they are always smiling because they know that every day they are helping their patients achieve better health, *without drugs*. It was so refreshing to see! I shook Gary's hand and sat down to explain the programs that I had been undergoing over the last six months. Again, I was curious to find out if Gary had ever heard of the Gerson program. *I was completely shocked at his answer!* Not only had he heard of it, but also many years earlier he actually worked at a similar clinic. He knew the Gerson programs like the back of his own hand. He told me many of the success stories he had seen in person at the clinic, and instantly I was re-energized to continue on my mission.

Gary began explaining his first program to me. It was called *live blood cell analysis.* It sounded unusual at first, but as he further explained the details, it was a simple concept to grasp. Basically, he would use a pin-sized needle to prick the end of my finger to obtain a small drop of blood. Next he would place the drop of blood onto a glass slide and then place the slide under a special microscope that would magnify my blood. The magnified blood picture would show up on a small television-sized monitor that we could view together. This is when Gary would give his expert diagnosis of my blood condition. It was truly amazing to see my blood cells up on the screen in live motion.

Using this program, you can see the condition of your blood with your very own eyes. An evaluation of your blood can tell if you need metabolic support and/or lifestyle changes to achieve a healthier system. This technique will reveal the status of your immune system, nutritional deficiencies, liver stress, toxins, risk factor of disease, candida, or parasites, and the condition of body systems.[1] Some of the findings can provide information about digestive efficiency, vitamin and mineral status, and much more. "Sticky" blood can cause fatigue and less oxygenation to the cells. Caffeine use, being around smokers, poor digestion, and even stress can be some of the contribution factors. The shapes and sizes of the red blood cells also reveals a great deal. For example, many irregular, fragmented cells can be an indicator of degenerative diseases. The white blood cells can be visually scanned and can give a good indication on the functioning of your immune system.[2] *Live cell microscopy is not a diagnostic procedure for any specific disease. It is best used as a screening test to help determine the optimal diet and natural program for a given individual with chronic illness, especially of the immune system.* Analysis of the blood by the microscope is as old as the practice of medicine itself. The main advantage of blood micros-copy is that many nutritional imbalances can be detected before standard chemical blood tests show any abnormalities. Health problems can then be prevented by early nutritional intervention.[3]

SAMPLE LIVE BLOOD CELL ANALYSIS PICTURES

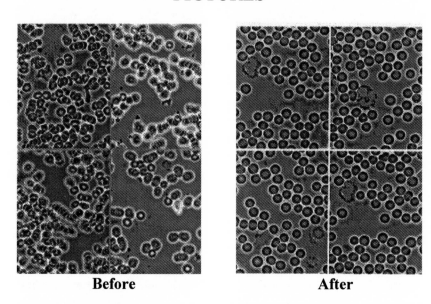

Before   **After**

Live cell analysis is a way of studying living whole blood cells under a specially adapted microscope...for arthritis patients, the testing can be particularly useful for viewing the distortions of red blood cells, which can indicate fatty acid deficiencies. Immune system analysis can be done by looking at the size, shape, and mobility of the white blood cells. Allergic status can be ascertained by the activity of the white blood cells that re-lease histamines. Live cell is a particularly useful tool because it helps patients visualize what is happening in their blood dur-ing the disease process; it also gives them immediate feedback on their efforts to improve health.

Let's look at some facts and principles of our blood. Our bodies are a miraculous network of 60,000 miles of blood vessels, with a heart muscle that pumps 55 million gallons of blood over the course of a lifetime to feed all 60 trillion cells in your body.[4] Amazingly, seven million new blood cells are produced every second. That's an incredible amount of new cells, and is a perfect example of how miraculous our bodies really are. Within the blood stream, normally the blood makes a complete circuit of the body every twenty-three seconds.[5] Further, physiology textbooks tell us that we make a new blood stream every twenty-eight days.[6] And another important fact is that our blood is over 90 percent water.[7] You might be wondering why I am telling you this; the reason is that you should know that the blood system is a very complex component of the body and *without healthy blood cells it is impossible to have good health.* Our blood is not just aimless liquid running throughout our bodies with no purpose. Blood is actually a type of connective tissue consisting of cells within a liquid, the blood plasma, which circulates through the heart and blood vessels. The blood carries vital nutrients to our other tissues and removes the waste products of their metabolism.[8] *Every tissue and organ in your body has to draw its replacement material from your blood stream.* This is true whether it is your eyes, muscles, heart, stomach, liver, or any organ of your body.[9]

Live blood cell analysis is the early key to recovery and provides a roadmap back to better health. Cells thrive when given these two conditions: proper nutrients and elimination of toxins.[10] *The cleaner your bloodstream, the healthier your body.* When you realize that every part of your body is bathed, washed, nourished, and oxygenated by your bloodstream around-the-clock, then you will understand the importance of having a clean "river of life". Improved diet, digestion, and absorption usually results in a quick improvement of the blood picture. As free radical levels decrease, consequent improvement in disease signs and symptoms usually follows soon after.[11] *If the healing capacity of the blood is now greater than the disease process, even chronic disease will quickly disappear.*[12] Taking this all into account, your blood is responsible for nourishing the energetic function and repair of every cell, organ, and system in your body. Your blood is part of your all-important immune system. White blood cells are its major workers. You can actually see if they are functioning properly. The bloodstream carries visible signs of how the other parts of your immune system are working, and indications of what's affecting them.[13]

Using this effective program, Gary and I worked together as a *"blood cleansing team"*. In the first few months, I would visit him every two weeks to see how my blood picture was progressing. After things were improving, I would only see him once a month. It was truly impressive to see my blood cells becoming cleaner after a few months on this program: my red blood cells were getting rounder; my white blood cells were functioning stronger; and with less waste material showing on the monitor, it showed that my digestion process was improving. It proved to me that by continuing to eat natural foods, juicing, and taking certain supplements that I could improve my blood picture, thus improving my overall health. This was just the first of Gary's programs. Now it was time for me to learn his next program on my continued mission to defeat my arthritis.

IRIS ANALYSIS (Iridology)

This program is the study of the iris of the eye, in order to diagnose genetic weaknesses and possibly halt future diseases. *Iridology is based on the assumption that every organ in the human body has a corresponding location within the iris, and that one can determine whether an organ is healthy or diseased by examining them.* Iris analysis was popularized in this country mainly through the work of Dr. Bernard Jensen, D.C. Dr. Jensen taught that the iris revealed tissue condition (levels of inflammation or degeneration) in the body. By knowing where the weak links are in the body, we can better determine what the probable underlying causes are of a person's health. The key is to remember that the presence of an iris sign is only an indication of a tendency, not an established fact.[14]

Fortunately for me, the great Dr. Bernard Jensen personally trained Gary in this technique. So not only did I have Gary on my health team, but I also had Dr. Jensen's expertise in my corner based on his teachings to Gary. Dr. Jensen has written many books on this subject, including *Science and Practice of Iridology Volumes I, II, and III, Iridology Simplified, What is Iridology?*, and *Visions of Health*. I knew Gary had studied and familiarized himself with these books, so I was extremely confident in his abilities to perform this technique. He was trained by Dr. Jensen, who is considered to be one of the geniuses of the natural health world. The more I learned about this program, the more fascinated I became. Everyone goes through life looking out at the world through their eyes and never once considering the possibility that our eyes are holding a key to our future. It is like we are all carrying a hidden secret within us and we don't even know it. Well, now it was time for me to unlock this secret, with Gary's help, to discover what my body could reveal about my health. Below are the standard eye charts we used to diagnose my iris signs.

STANDARD IRIDOLOGY CHARTS

Right Eye Chart and Corresponding Body Areas

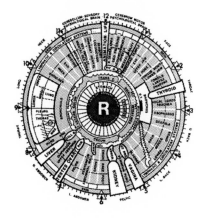 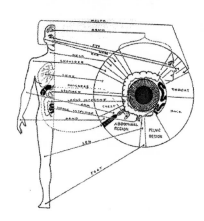

Left Eye Chart and Corresponding Body Areas

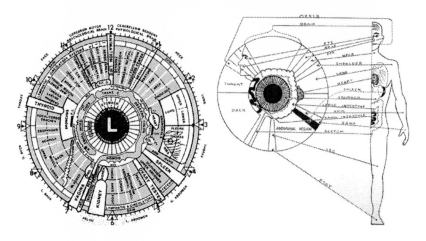

One hundred and fifty years ago it was discovered that each area of the body has a representative area in the iris of the eye. In effect, the iris works like a color television screen, the cameras being found in every cell of the body. By looking in the iris, some of the early preconditions of disease can be seen.[15]

The program determined that my iris signs pointed to weaknesses in my kidneys and adrenal glands, and poor digestion. This didn't surprise me too much, considering that Dr. Baird also found these to be my weak points using her kinesiology testing. So my goal was to focus on using vitamins and herbs that would strengthen and rebuild these organs. So far I had learned two new amazing programs from Gary, and now it was time to move on to the next one. I felt like an undercover agent discovering all these non-traditional programs. *The average medical doctor has never been trained in these natural programs; therefore they have no understanding on how effective they can be at healing the body.* I guess, in a strange way, my health mission was an adventure as well as a cure.

CYCLE DETOXIFICATION PROGRAM

The human body has many organs that work hard every day to help keep the body clean and healthy. It is of great importance that we eat the right foods to keep them that way. Unfortunately in today's busy society, it is hard to find the time or the place to accomplish this goal. That is the reason we may need to take certain supplements to compensate for this unhealthy eating and lifestyle choices. One valuable lesson Gary taught me is that there are certain formulas that can help you in the task of keeping these organs functioning properly. Using a cycle detoxification program, I was able to take certain formulas to accomplish this goal.

Remember in the detoxification section of chapter 4, I talked about the car versus the body analogies. I mentioned how the different organs, or filters, perform the job of detoxifying our bodies. If we don't keep these organs healthy, the body will break down just like a car. Well, that concept applies directly to these formulas. I learned that using these formulas in different cycles could help my body become stronger and healthier. One rule that Gary mentioned is that you shouldn't try to detoxify and strengthen all your organs at once. This would be overwhelming on the body, since detoxifying takes a great deal of the body's energy. It should be done in a slow, gradual process, focusing on one or two of these systems at a time. That's why it's called cycle detoxification. Personally, I started with the colon cleanse formula for a month, and then moved on to another formula and focused on it for a month. I would rotate through these until I finished with all of them. Then I would start the process over again to strengthen and cleanse these organ systems as much as possible. As I became stronger, I then used these formulas in various combinations to achieve higher success. Below, I have listed some of the important formulas and their ingredients that I used throughout my entire program.

Adrenal Gland Support
Contains adrenal tissue, spleen tissue, zinc, pantothenic acid, vitamin B-6, niacinamide, riboflavin, thiamine, vitamin C, and vitamin A.

Blood Cleanse Formula
Contains red clover, chaparral, licorice root, peach bark, stillingia, prickly ash, burdock root, pokeroot, Oregon grape, and buckthorn.

Colon Cleanse Formula
Contains oat fiber, black currant fiber, psyllium, carrageenan, fenugreek, fennel, ginger, rosemary, peppermint, flax, lecithin, acidophilus, and an enzyme blend.

Gall Bladder Formula
Contains Oregon grape root, ginger root, cramp bark, fennel seeds, peppermint leaves, and wild yam root.

Joint Formula
Contains bromelain, yarrow flowers, hydrangea root, capsicum fruit, yucca root, valerian root, horsetail herb, white willow bark, celery seed, burdock root, alfalfa herb, slippery elm bark, black cohosh root, and sarsaparilla root.

Kidney Cleanse Formula
Contains parsley, uva ursi, marshmallow, juniper, buchu, cleavers, corn silk, dandelion, yarrow, and hydrangea.

Liver Cleanse Formula
Contains dandelion root, barberry bark, milk thistle, burdock, rose hips, fennel seeds, horseradish root, parsley herb, and red beetroot.

7

Dr. Terry Pfau
Homeopathic Help from
Las Vegas

"I believe the doctor of the future will be a teacher as well as a physician. His real job will be to teach people how to be healthy."

---D.C. Jarvis, M.D.

It was now May of 1994. I had been using the natural programs for about nine months, and my progress was amazing. On the same 1 to 10 scale as before, I would say I was now about a 7 ½. It had been about three months since I had last seen Dr. Baird, so I decided to schedule another appointment with her. I knew it would be nice to get a checkup to determine how my body was progressing. I drove to her office, and just as I imagined, her energy level was incredible and of course she still had that great big smile. I explained the experience I'd had the last few months working with Gary, and thanked her again for introducing me to him.

As she was doing her adjustments on me, we talked about our current lives and what was new and exciting. I told her that my parents were planning on moving to Las Vegas, and that they were curious if she knew any natural doctors that they could visit out there. Both my father and mother had been to Dr. Baird with great results, so they were firm believers in natural programs as well. She did indeed know a doctor in the Las Vegas area, and gave me his name and number. She had worked with this doctor in the past, and felt that he was very qualified. She also felt that he could not only help my parents, but also be a great addition to my program. At this point my life was going to change for the better once again.

Dr. Baird asked me if I had heard of homeopathy. I told her that I had come across it a few times in my readings and research, but had never used it. She felt that this would be another great program for me to incorporate into my overall program to help defeat my arthritis. The doctor she mentioned was Dr. Terry Pfau, and he was an osteopathic physician (D.O.) and a homeopathic medical doctor (H.M.D.). He was a highly trained physician who not only specialized in homeopathy, but also looked at the body as a "whole person" approach to medicine. *Instead of just treating specific symptoms or illnesses, he assessed the overall health of his patients, including their lifestyles and home and work environments.* I knew that I would be traveling to Las Vegas soon, so I was looking forward to meeting with Dr. Pfau. My next mission was to learn another amazing program.

HOMEOPATHIC PROGRAM

I was in Las Vegas the next month, visiting my parents in their new home. I set up an appointment with Dr. Pfau to find out more about his program and how it could improve my condition. I arrived at my appointment, and the first thing I noticed about him was that he was very deliberate and observant with his actions. Even though he was young – probably just in his mid-thirties - he appeared to be very wise, as though he had the experience of many lifetimes. He reminded me of the expression, "The older you get, the wiser you become". We sat down and talked about his program and how it might be able to help me. I explained all the programs that I had done up to that point, and he was in complete agreement with my approach. I knew that, once again, I had another team member in my overall quest.

So what is homeopathy? Homeopathy is a low-cost, non-toxic system of medicine used by hundreds of millions of people worldwide. *It is particularly effective in treating chronic illnesses that fail to respond to conventional treatment, and is also a superb method of care for minor conditions such as the common cold and flu.*[1] It is a system based on principles that have not changed for nearly 200 years. This consistency in adhering to healing principles has allowed homeopathy to establish itself as one of the most integrated, complete systems of healing. It originated in Germany, and is now widely practiced throughout the world. It conforms to a law of healing known as the "law of similars." This law of healing was formally established and developed by Samuel Hahnemann, a German physician who lived between 1764 and 1843.

Homeopathy is a form of treatment that gently nudges the body toward a healthier state.[2] *Homeopathic remedies neither cover up nor destroy diseases by themselves. Rather, they stimulate the body's own natural defenses to rid it of the disease.* Therefore, they do not cause adverse side effects, as some powerful drugs do. Homeopathic remedies are completely safe.[3]

Some of the main benefits of Homeopathy:

- Treats the Whole Person
- A Gentle System of Healing
- Very Effective in Both Acute and Chronic Conditions
- Remove Long-Standing Physical Problems
- Increase Overall Energy
- Non Toxic with No Side Effects
- Economical and Less Expensive than Drugs

After I explained the other programs I had been using to Dr. Pfau, it was time for him to explain his program to me. The program in itself is the homeopathic medicine, but to determine which homeopathic remedy is right for the patient is where the skill is required. He asked me questions concerning my complete lifestyle, such as: my sleeping habits, eating habits, work habits, my reaction to stress, my body weight fluctuations, energy levels, and of course my arthritis conditions. He also asked me questions that were specific to my arthritis: where was the pain the worst, was the pain worse in the mornings or evenings, and was the skin hot to the touch or just swollen? I knew there was a reason that Dr. Pfau was very methodical in his actions. He needed to be as observant as possible to make the important decision on which homeopathic remedy would be right for me. This wasn't as easy as going to the health food store and picking one out from the shelf. It had to be the exact remedy that would get to the root of my problem. *I knew I was dealing with an expert!*

The appointment lasted at least an hour and a half. As I mentioned before, these natural health doctors really take their time with their patients, to get to know them and make sure they are giving the right advice. Dr. Pfau made his decision on which remedy was right for me, and it was time for me to start this new program. I walked out of his office with my remedy in hand and felt very confident that I had just found another piece of the puzzle to defeat my arthritis once and for all.

I returned to California and began taking the homeopathic remedy. Within a few days, things took a turn for the worse - or so I thought. The pains that I used to have in my right toes, left ankle, and lower back all came back. I was shocked that after nine months of working with my programs that the pain could come back that quickly. I called Dr. Pfau immediately and told him something was terribly wrong, and that I was in pain again. In his normal, well thought out, calm manner, he said that everything was okay. He explained that healing the body works in different stages, almost as if there are multiple layers. He further explained that people who are being treated with homeopathic medicine for a chronic disease sometimes experience a temporary exacerbation in their symptoms as the body's defenses are being stimulated. He taught me that this was a good sign, and an indication that my body was healing itself. But he also explained that using a remedy with too high a potency can actually over-stimulate these symptoms and aggravate your condition. This is especially true in a person who has been weakened by their disease, or when the disease has been suppressed for long periods of time by traditional medicines. This was the reason that finding the exact homeopathic remedy was of the utmost importance, and also the reason that I was using an expert like Dr. Pfau. In the words of Dana Ullman, M.P.H, in her article, *A Modern Understanding of Homeopathic Medicine*, "Homeopathic medicines are prescribed to aid the person in its highly sophisticated efforts to heal. Inherent in the homeopathic approach is a basic respect for the body's wisdom; it is thus no wonder that it is a safer medicine."[4]

So I continued on with the remedy, knowing that it would work as long as I was patient and let it run its course. This was very difficult, because it felt like I was moving backwards in my program in which I had worked so hard. But I had to think long-term. My body responded within the next week as the pain disappeared. My checkups with Dr. Pfau were a little unusual. Since I lived California and he was in Las Vegas, we would have phone consultations to determine my status. Together we would discuss my overall health to determine if I was still on the correct remedy or if another one was necessary. It all turned out just fine, and through this I learned that homeopathic remedies work extremely well. They had proven to be effective at relieving disorders due to their ability to remove deep-seated toxins from the body.[5] I also knew that my body had just reached a higher plateau of health, and that I was that much closer to stopping my arthritis forever.

Effective treatment with homeopathic medicine is possible for the vast numbers of people with chronic illness today. Real cure is possible with homeopathy. In 1980, the *British Journal of Clinical Pharmacology* published a double-blind study that showed the impressive effects of homeopathic medicines on people suffering from autoimmune arthritis. Researchers found that 82% of those given homeopathic medicines experienced a positive type of health benefit.[6] We all know that staying healthy is a long-term objective. The long-term benefit of homeopathy to the patient is that it not only alleviates the presenting symptoms, but it re-establishes internal order at the deepest levels and thereby provides a lasting cure.[7]

8

Other Natural Supplements Immune System Boosters

"I believe that you can, by taking some simple and inexpensive measures, extend your life and years of well-being. My most important recommendation is that you take vitamins every day to optimum amounts, to supplement the vitamins you receive in your food."
   ---Linus Pauling, Ph.D., Two-time Nobel Prize Laureate

Throughout my entire program I was amazed with the number of natural supplements available that had positive health benefits. It seemed like every health book or health article I read had proven research on supplements that improved certain health conditions. Hopefully you noticed that I said *"proven research."* The reason I did this, and the reason I am providing proven research throughout this book, is so you understand that natural programs are real. These programs are not quackery like many medical doctors want us to believe. Since I was on a mission to improve my health to the highest plateau to defeat my arthritis, of course I was going to use every means possible to accomplish this goal. So that's exactly what I did. I had a full arsenal of supplements to choose from to help in my fight. Keep in mind that these supplements are not just for arthritis, but also for many other degenerative diseases and for overall better health. In fact, recent studies in distinguished professional publications, such as the *New England Journal of Medicine* and the *Journal of the American Medical Association*, report that vitamins and minerals appear to have a protective effect against certain diseases, including cancer, diabetes, high blood pressure, heart disease, and osteoporosis.[1] Also, a twenty-four year nutritional study by the University of Southern California on 11,384 men and women revealed that not only did the daily consumption of vitamins and minerals cut the death rate in half, but it also reduced the death rate for cancer and heart disease tenfold.[2]

Try not to become overwhelmed by all these supplements. I can assure you that I didn't take all of these at the same time. I used these supplements in different combinations to determine which ones provided me with the greatest results. Remember, healing the body is a slow process and shouldn't be rushed. One thing is for sure; I will be taking these for the rest of my life.

MULTIVITAMIN/MINERAL SUPPLEMENT

I would have to recommend that a multivitamin/mineral supplement is the most important one to begin with in your program. It protects you from any missing links you may have in your diet and the foods that you are eating. Be careful, though; there are different kinds on the shelves, and it is hard to know which one is the correct one to buy. For example, you should buy vitamins from a health food store that contain "whole food" ingredients, and not the synthetic substitutes commonly found in grocery and drugstore supplements. These synthetic substitutes are foreign substances that cannot be properly metabolized by the body, and can eventually cause toxic buildup.[3] *Synthetic vitamins are vitamins produced in laboratories from isolated chemicals that mirror their counterparts found in nature. Natural vitamins are derived from food sources.*[4] Author and nutrition expert Patrick Quillin, Ph.D., R.D., C.N.S., explains, "I generally discourage the use of cheap multivitamins found in the grocery store or pharmacy."[5] Also, remember to avoid any multivitamins with artificial colors such as FD&C yellow #5 (tartrazine). These artificial ingredients can interfere with the body's metabolism of certain vitamins, such as vitamin B_6. Make sure the label states that the formula contains no corn, wheat, soy, milk, yeast, starch or lactose. Also, capsules are generally better absorbed than tablets.[6]

Keep in mind that this supplement should be taken with meals. The reason for this is that vitamins and minerals perform synergistically with one another.[7] That means they work together as a team. Taking supplements with meals helps to assure a supply of other nutrients needed for better assimilation.[8] I think most people would be surprised at how many people are missing certain nutrients in their diets. Statistics tell us that more than 60 percent of us are deficient in vitamin B_6, magnesium, chromium, calcium, iron, zinc, and fiber.[9] So make sure that this supplement is on top of your shopping list.

ACIDOPHILUS

There are more than 400 different kinds of bacteria that live in our gastrointestinal tract. Acidophilus, also known as probiotics, is very important in protecting and adding beneficial bacteria to this digestive tract. The body depends on these beneficial bacteria to stop invading pathogens from colonizing in the intestine, produce and regulate vitamin levels, stimulate digestive function, remove accumulated toxins, and maintain chemical and hormonal balance, as well as produce lactase and other antibacterial substances. With the proliferation of preservatives, additives, high-fat diets, alcohol, birth control pills, and stress in our society, the result can be poor intestinal flora. Antibiotic drugs are especially damaging to intestinal flora and kill all kinds of bacteria, both good and bad. According to S.K. Dash, Ph.D., expert in the field of probiotics, "The benefits of acidophilus are that it produces B vitamins, produces lactase enzymes and helps digest lactose, helps digest food, prevents bad breath, and inhibits and reduces candidiasis (yeast infection)."[10] I have recommended this supplement to a few friends who have had stomach issues for years, and they said that within a few weeks it worked wonders for them and they wish they had known about it much sooner.

ALPHA-LIPOIC ACID

This supplement is one of the best antioxidants known to man. According to Lester Packer, Ph.D., a molecular and cellular biologist at the University of California, Berkeley, "People tap the full antioxidant benefits of alpha-lipoic acid only when they take it as a supplement." *Dr. Packer, one of the top antioxidant researchers in the world, is clearly excited about the nutrient.* In a recent interview, he politely sidestepped questions about the antioxidants that he takes, but he unabashedly admitted that he does take alpha-lipoic acid supplements. Alpha-lipoic acid is unique for this reason: it's a major player in antioxidant synergism— what Packer prefers to call the body's "antioxidant network." Alpha-lipoic acid helps the body recycle and renew vitamins C and E, Co-Q10 and glutathione—thus extending their metabolic lifetimes. Packer has at various times described it as the "metabolic," "universal," and "ideal" antioxidant. Coming from a leading scientist, such words are particularly meaningful. According to Packer, alpha-lipoic acid supplements are easily absorbed and may be preferable to the major dietary source of the nutrient, which is red meat.[11]

What makes alpha-lipoic acid so special as an antioxidant is that it helps deactivate a wide array of *fat and water-soluble free radicals* in the body. In particular, it may help protect the genetic material, DNA. It is also important because it works closely with vitamins C and E and other antioxidants, "recycling" them and thus making them much more effective.[12] If you have arthritis, then it is of special value. Arthritis, psoriasis, and asthma: all of these conditions involve inflammation. By enhancing the effects of other antioxidants, alpha-lipoic acid raises the body's levels of natural anti-inflammatory prostaglandins and decreases the levels of inflammatory prostaglandins. The result is often a marked improvement of these conditions.[13] Since we know that the liver is so important to our health, keeping it functioning at an optimum level is vital. Jesse Stoff, M.D., director of IntegaMed in Tucson, AZ, says, "Alpha-lipoic acid is one of the supplements that should be taken, especially for chronic liver inflammation."[14] So we can sum it up by saying that alpha-lipoic acid is an exciting addition to the list of nutrients and herbs that can treat disease in a safer and more natural way, and help you become healthier.[15]

APPLE CIDER VINEGAR AND HONEY

This is an old wives' tale, but I think taking apple cider vinegar and honey with meals is very important for a few reasons. *First, digestion might be the most important function that the body performs* (I will discuss digestion in more detail in chapter 11). According to D.C. Jarvis, M.D, in his book, *Arthritis and Folk Medicine*, we know that vinegar, honey, and water during meals greatly improves digestion and brings about a disappearance of heartburn and gas formation in the stomach after eating.[16] Secondly, we have already discussed the importance of the blood to our health. It's true that vinegar and water at each meal increases the amount of hemoglobin in the blood, which means that more red blood cells carrying hemoglobin are present.[17] More red blood cells equals a better quality of blood, which results in a healthier body. And last but not least, one of the symptoms of arthritis is buildup of acid crystals in the joints. If we can lessen this buildup, it will improve the arthritis. As Paul and Patricia Bragg state, "Two teaspoons of organic apple cider vinegar will fight the buildup of uric acid crystals that have a tendency to form in our body over the years. These eventually cause disorders such as bursitis and other joint problems."[18] So give it a try - it tastes pretty good, and I feel that it was another helping hand in my overall success.

BROMELAIN

I can't say enough about the benefit of taking bromelain if you have any type of inflammation disorder, like arthritis. More than 200 scientific papers have been written about bromelain since it was first introduced as a health-boosting substance in 1957.

Much of the research has focused on anti-inflammatory effects. Whether you have a sprained ankle, a nasty bruise, sinusitis, or any other type of inflammation, bromelain may help you heal faster.[19] It is extracted from the stem of ripe pineapples, and it mainly helps to reduce swelling and break up some of the antigen-antibody complexes involved in autoimmune reactions.[20] Not only would I take this in supplemental form, but I would also juice pineapples so that I would benefit from fresh bromelain.

To support this amazing supplement even further, Dr. Hans Nieper, a world-renowned physician, reported that bromelain was slowly and steadily effective in lowering blood pressure and was "one of the most effective anti-arthritics." It stops platelet aggregation—the stickiness of the blood.[21] And in another study, "Bromelain inhibits the release of certain inflammation-causing chemicals," explains Alan L. Miller, N.D., technical advisor for Thorne Research in Sandpoint, Idaho, and senior editor of *Alternative Medicine Review*.[22] Clearly, this supplement should not be left out of your diet by anyone who is suffering with arthritis or any other kind of inflammation.

CHERRY JUICE

There is a form of arthritis called gout. It is a type of arthritis that mostly affects men age 40 and older. It is nearly always associated with an abnormally high concentration of uric acid in the blood. Uric acid is a byproduct of certain foods, so gout is closely related to diet. Gout has been called the "rich man's disease," since it is associated with too much alcohol and rich foods such as meat, white flour, sugar, cakes and pies. Avoiding these will help greatly. Cherries contain flavonoid compounds that may lower uric acid and reduce inflammation. So, taking a cherry juice supplement, eating cherries, or drinking natural cherry juice will definitely lower uric acid levels and reduce the pain associated with gout.

COD LIVER OIL (Omega-3s)

I know many of you reading this are saying, "Oh no, not cod liver oil; it tastes so bad." Don't worry; I have good news for you because there is an alternative. You can purchase flavored cod liver oil, or even buy it in capsule form so that you don't have to taste it at all. Personally, I buy the mint-flavored oil, and that seems to work well for me. But regardless of taste, this is one supplement that you can't do without.

In his popular book, *The Omega Rx Zone*, Dr. Barry Sears talks about the benefits of the oil, claiming that "consuming calibrated amounts of high-dose fish oil will help treat chronic disease, improve athletic performance, and promote emotional well-being."[23] This is a strong statement, considering that Dr. Sears, Ph.D., is a widely published scientist and researcher who holds thirteen U.S. patents. In addition to this, in a Cardiff research study, Professor Bruce Caterson of the School of Biomedicine at Cardiff University looked at the effect of Omega-3 fatty acids (the main component of cod liver oil) and found that the supplement *can delay or even reverse the destruction of joint cartilage and inflammatory pain associated with arthritic disease*. And to comment on that statement, Fergus Logan, chief executive of the Arthritis Research Campaign, said: "Thanks to Professor Caterson, we now know precisely what cod liver oil can do, where it can help and how it helps treat the body."[24]

The benefits of cod liver oil come from the omega-3s. Omega-3s are natural blood thinners that prevent blood clots that can lead to heart attack or stroke. They also protect against certain forms of cancer. Animal studies show that they can decrease the number and size of tumors. They are also anti-inflammatory and are useful in the treatment of arthritis.[25] I believe that if you want to help yourself and help defeat your arthritis or any other inflammatory condition, you should, without a doubt, be taking cod liver oil (omega-3s). Otherwise, you will be fighting an uphill battle. That's how important it is in the fight against arthritis.

DMSO

We don't hear much about this persecuted product because it cannot be patented, since it is made from a natural source. *And even though it's been proven to work in more than 3000 independent studies that all firmly establish its power and safety, the FDA will not allow doctors to prescribe it.*[26] This is a shame, because I can fully attest that it works for arthritis pain and swelling. DMSO has remarkable therapeutic properties, especially for the healing of injuries. Applying DMSO on sprained ankles, pulled muscles, dislocated joints, and even at the site of simple fractures can virtually eliminate pain. It also promotes immune system activity.[27]

The fact remains that this product works to restore function in illnesses like arthritis and immune system disease, and it is very helpful in acute inflammatory pain syndromes.[28] Stephen Edelson, MD, F.A.A.F.P., F.A.A.E.M., who practices medicine at the Environmental and Preventive Health Center of Atlanta, has used DMSO extensively for 4 years. He says, "We use it intravenously as well as locally. We use it for all sorts of inflammatory conditions, from people with rheumatoid arthritis to people with chronic low back inflammatory-type symptoms, silicon immune toxicity syndromes, or any kind of autoimmune process."[29] In yet another powerhouse study, it was found that DMSO reduces swelling because of its powerful anti-inflammatory properties. It is versatile and truly amazing, especially in treating arthritis. Studies have shown that this exceptionally safe substance increases blood flow and oxygen availability to the injured area."[30]

FOOD ENZYMES

The importance of maintaining high levels of food enzymes in our bodies cannot be overemphasized. Our bodies have over 80,000 enzyme systems, each with a specific function: from determining the color of our eyes, to aiding the digestion of food, and even controlling the movement of the retina as we speak. Enzymes are found in *live raw foods only*, which are fruits, vegetables, nuts, and seeds. Cooking kills enzymes. Prolonged heat above 118 degrees Fahrenheit also destroys enzymes in food. Three minutes in boiling water destroys the enzymes; pasteurization destroys 80 to 95 percent; and baking, frying, broiling, stewing and canning destroy 100 percent. Nature designed food with sufficient enzymes within it to digest that food when it is eaten. When enzymes are destroyed by cooking or other processing, ingesting that food triggers the body's immune system to respond.[31] So the only way to get food enzymes is to eat raw foods, or the other easy alternative is take food enzyme supplements.

The first major scientific paper on enzymes was published in 1940, by Dr. Edward Howell, in *The Journal of the American Association for Medico-Physical Research*. Dr. Howell is formally recognized as the discoverer of the vital role of enzymes in human nutrition. *He pioneered more than 50 years of research and scientific experimentation with overwhelming evidence indicating that the primary cause of degenerative disease in humans is enzyme deficiencies.*[32] Dr. Howell called enzymes the "sparks of life." Life as we know it could not exist without the action of enzymes, even in the presence of sufficient amounts of vitamins, minerals, water, and other nutrients.[33] Dr. Howell, interviewed in the compilation of his enzyme research, *Food Enzymes for Health Longevity*, summarized the following in relation to animal models: "Diets deficient in enzymes cause a 30 percent reduction in life-span." He recommends including raw foods in the modern diet, but recognizes that this would not overcome the current enzyme drain. He states, "The only solution is to take capsules of food enzymes."[34]

In a statement by Majid Ali, M.D., and author of the *Life Span Library* of books, "Enzymes are molecules that give living things the quality of life."[35] Clinical experience shows that enzymes work well as a digestive aid, help to initiate tissue repair, and help restore the balance of GI flora.[36] And that leads us to the reason enzyme supplements are so important. Supplemental food enzymes serve two functions: *eaten with food, they aid digestion by ensuring the complete metabolization of fat, proteins and carbohydrates; ingested on an empty stomach for blood detoxification, they are absorbed into the blood and clean long-term resid-*

ual food particles.[37] In my program, I was obtaining these enzymes by eating fresh fruit, juicing fresh vegetables, and also by taking the enzyme supplements daily. I wanted to make sure that I had an abundant level of enzymes available for my body to use wisely. It was essential!

GLUCOSAMINE/CHONDROITIN SULFATES

Glucosamine and chondroitin sulfate are substances found naturally in the body. Glucosamine is a form of amino sugar that plays a role in cartilage formation and repair. Chondroitin sulfate is part of a large protein molecule that promotes water retention and elasticity in cartilage. Together they can help protect and even repair the joints. According to Michael T. Murray, N.D., "Glucosamine sulfate has been the topic of over 300 research studies and more than 20 double-blind studies. It has been used by millions of people throughout the world, and is an approved drug for osteoarthritis in over 70 countries."[38]

In their successful book, *The Arthritis Cure*, Jason Theodosakis, M.D., Brenda Adderly, M.H.A., and Barry Fox, Ph.D., go into great detail about the use of glucosamine and chondroitin. They state, "Glucosamine not only successfully quells pain and other symptoms of osteoarthritis, it does so more effectively than ibuprofen, the active ingredient in Advil, Motrin, Nuprin, and other popular arthritis remedies."[39] They further note that "chondroitin sulfates also help prevent premature breakdown of cartilage in two ways: they stop the naturally occurring enzymes from going haywire and actually 'chewing' up cartilage, and they inhibit other enzymes from shutting off the flow of nutrients to the cartilage."[40] In another popular book, *Preventing and Reversing Arthritis Naturally*, Raquel Martin and Karen Romano, R.N., D.C., state, "Chondroitin helps restore collagen and proteoglycans in injured joints. It also stimulates an amino acid, hyaluronan, and protects the building blocks of cartilage cells."[41] With these comments, we can see that each of these sulfates is highly effective in the fight against joint pain.

But using these supplements in combination is even more effective. Together, glucosamine and chondroitin increase production of collagen, the framework of cartilage; slow certain enzymes that prematurely destroy cartilage; block enzymes that interfere with the transfer of nutrients to the cartilage; and increase the production of proteoglycans, the molecules that help cartilage stay wet and healthy.[42] And to further support this, an article published in the *Journal of the American Medical Association*, analyzed data from six studies on glucosamine and nine on chondroitin published between 1966 and 1999. Overall, the research showed moderate to significant benefits on pain and mobility, compared to a placebo, in patients with arthritis in the hip or knee. There were no serious side effects.[43] The benefits of these supplements are so overwhelming that they are an absolute must as an addition to your daily regimen.

GRAPE SEED EXTRACT (OPCs)

Grape seed extract is a powerful antioxidant that can reduce the damage done by free radicals, strengthen and repair connective tissue, and promote enzyme activity. Grape seed extract (also known as Oligomeric ProanthoCyanidins, or OPCs) can also help moderate allergic and inflammatory responses by reducing histamine production. When OPCs extracted from grape seeds are taken as nutritional supplements, they turn into highly potent antioxidants and are superior cell and tissue protectors. OPCs possess a unique strong affinity to bond with collagen. Also, OPCs strengthen and rebuild elastin in the body that bonds with vascular walls.[44]

This potent bioflavonoid extracted from the seeds of grapes is so essential to our existence that it should be considered a vitamin because our bodies cannot make it. *It has been shown to be 20 times more potent than vitamin C and 50 times more potent than vitamin E as an antioxidant.* It has a selective affinity for the connective tissue of the body. It strengthens and protects collagen and elastin fibers of the connective tissue found in the skin, heart, blood vessels, joints, gums, mucous membranes, and cell membranes from the effects of free radicals.[45] This ability of grape seed extract to stabilize and protect collagen and elastin within joints has demonstrated remarkable effects in the relief of pain and inflammation associated with arthritis.[46]

I had a friend ask me for advice on the topic of varicose veins, and if there was a supplement that could help his mother with this condition. I knew that grape seed extract was perfect for this kind of situation, so that's what I recommended. She took the supplement, and after just one month she noticed a remarkably difference in the condition of her varicose veins. They were less swollen and less raised above the surface of the skin. This is a known fact with grape seed extract. In fact, many major clinical studies have shown marked benefits in treating circulation problems involving venous insufficiency, varicose veins, capillary fragility, and disorders of the retina, including macular degeneration and diabetic retinopathy. In one study with healthy volunteers, 200 mg per day significantly improved visual function within six weeks.[47]

KELP

Kelp, a highly nutrient-rich type of sea plant, contains over 75 minerals and trace elements. Because all of these minerals are present in seawater, kelp acts like a sponge that soaks them up and converts them into an organic form the body can safely absorb. Unlike synthetic vitamin and mineral supplements, the minerals and trace elements in kelp are organically bound, which make them totally absorbable. Kelp is one of nature's most complete sources of these vital nutrients.

One of the nutrients that kelp is particularly rich in is iodine. Iodine is very important for the thyroid gland to function properly, as this gland is an important regulator of metabolism and weight. I know that Dr. Max Gerson was a firm believer in the use of iodine supplementation. He recommended using a lugol solution as the source of iodine. I was having trouble finding this solution, so I decided to use kelp tablets instead. Regardless of which one you decide to use, they are both great for the immune system and add to the arsenal of supplements that are available for our bodies.

MSM

This is one supplement that you may have heard about on the news a few years back. It was in 1999, and it aired on *CBS 2 News Special Assignment*. It was an interview done by Michael Tuck with the famous actor James Coburn. It was called *"Coburn's Magic Bullet"* and it was all about the fact that Mr. Coburn had suffered with rheumatoid arthritis for over 30 years. But all of a sudden he started taking MSM, and the results were outstanding. *His pain almost completely disappeared.* In 1990, he could barely walk because of rheumatoid arthritis. He states in the interview, "I was really sick with it for a long time—until I stopped seeing doctors. *Doctors want to give you drugs and keep you on them. I wanted to get to the root of the problem."*[48] So he started reading everything he could find on rheumatoid arthritis, went on a 15-day fast and did colon-cleansing daily. He says, "That started the cure. It's an insidious immune disease. The body works against itself."[49] Finally, Coburn found MSM. He says "It really, really does the job. It's non-toxic, and helps stop the pain."[50]

Dr. Ronald M. Lawrence, who is the Assistant Clinical Professor of the UCLA School of Medicine, Founding Member of the American Association for the Study of Pain, and the American Association for the Study of Headaches, said, "Many of my rheumatoid arthritis patients report a rapid and substantial relief from symptoms. I find this amazing supplement helps even the most severe conditions."[51] One of the reasons is that MSM has been shown to allow for better passage of water and nutrients into the cells; this process also allows for wastes and toxins to properly flow out of the cells.[52]

And as if that's not enough proof, Dr. Earl Mindell, Ph.D., professor of Nutritional Studies at Pacific Western University and one of America's top health writers, said, "People with arthritis report substantial and long-lasting relief while supplementing MSM in their diet. MSM has also demonstrated a remarkable ability to reduce the incidence of, or entirely eliminate, soreness, leg and back cramps."[53] MSM is truly a miracle for pain relief. Professor Ronald Lawrence, M.D., Ph.D., conducted a double-blind study and reported that patients suffering from degenerative arthritis who took MSM on a daily basis experienced as much as 80 percent pain relief.[54] I highly recommend that when buying this product you look for the "Lignisul MSM" type. It is the first brand of MSM specifically developed as a pure food-grade nutritional supplement for human consumption. Plus, this type is a non-animal-based supplement derived from pine trees. And unlike most forms of MSM, including those imported from China, it's natural, not synthetic. The bottom line here is that MSM is a supplement that *works for arthritis pain.*

POTASSIUM

With the high sodium foods that are typical of the American diet, it is extremely important to get extra potassium. The potassium-sodium balance is very delicate in the body, and the goal of everyone should be to have a higher intake of potassium versus sodium on a daily basis. This is a mineral that Dr. Max Gerson was adamant about within his book, *A Cancer Therapy: Results of Fifty Cases.*

According to Thomas Pickering, M.D., D.Phil., FRCP, and Director of Integrative and Behavioral Cardiology Program of the Cardiovascular Institute at Mount Sinai School of Medicine in New York, "There is a steady, increasing body of evidence that a high-potassium intake may help not only to control blood pressure, but also to prevent its consequences, such as strokes and heart attacks."[55] "The higher the potassium and the less of the sodium is one way to have a more balanced blood pressure," says Ray W. Gifford, Jr., M.D., director of regional health affairs with the Cleveland (Ohio) Clinic Foundation. He goes on to say, "It may very well be beneficial as a non-pharmacological remedy. A potassium supplement may be very helpful."[56]

"High potassium foods help lower blood pressure, but potassium exhibits additional powers to prevent stroke directly regardless of blood pressure," says University of Minnesota hypertension expert Dr. Louis Tobian, Jr. His theory is that extra potassium keeps artery walls elastic and functioning normally, thus immunizing blood vessels against damage from high blood pressure.[57] In tests at Temple University School of Medicine, ten men with normal blood pressure ate a potassium-adequate diet, then a potassium-restricted diet, each for nine days. Deprived of potassium, the men experienced an average jump in arterial pressure of 4.1 points—up from 90.0 to 95. Their blood pressure shot even higher when the men's diets were loaded with sodium. Thus, potassium also helps keep a high-sodium diet in check, said the study's senior author, G. Gopal Krishna, M.D. He theorizes that too little potassium leads to sodium retention, which over time may trigger high blood pressure.[58] Yet again, here is another supplement that helps the overall health of the body to win the battle against arthritis and other diseases.

VITAMIN C

Now I know that everyone has heard of vitamin C. It's probably the most popular supplement on the market. The thing that doesn't make any sense is that the RDA (recommended dietary allowance) for vitamin C is set at only 60 mg. Yet, according to the genius and two-time Nobel laureate, Linus Pauling, Ph.D., "take vitamin C every day, 6,000 mg to 18,000 mg. Do not miss a single day."[59] This is a huge discrepancy of over 100 times more than the RDA. Something is definitely wrong with these numbers. I will have to take sides with the two-time Nobel prize winner and take the higher levels of vitamin C daily. In fact, over the last ten years I have taken between 2000 – 6000 mg daily to make sure that my body is fully enriched.

In medical literature, it is described as virtually non-toxic. Human beings have been given as much as 150 grams (150,000 mg), one-third of a pound, of vitamin C by injection or intravenous infusion without any serious side effects.[60] Vitamin C is no more toxic than ordinary sugar, less toxic than common salt, and far less toxic than aspirin or other drugs. There is no reported case of death or severe illness of any person from ingesting too large an amount of vitamin C.[61] A study done at Arizona State University showed that high doses of vitamin C, 2,000 mg daily for two weeks, can significantly lower histamine levels and may help the immune system fight against infection[62] And according to Gary Null, Ph.D., "The recommended dosage is 1,000 mg to 20,000 mg a day, depending on the state of your health and immune system."[63] So when I hear people say that we only need 60 mg a day, I feel for them, because they are listening to the RDA guidelines and are cheating their bodies of its full health potential (I will explain the RDA levels later in Chapter 11).

According to researchers at the USDA Human Nutrition Research Center on Aging at Tufts University, "Vitamin C may help prevent coronary artery disease. Researchers studied blood vitamin C levels of men and women ranging in age from 20 to 100. Those with the highest blood levels of vitamin C had the highest levels of HDL or good cholesterol, and those with the lowest C levels had the lowest levels of good cholesterol. High vitamin C levels were also associated with lower blood pressure."[64] Vitamin C is also involved with many other important bodily functions, like collagen formation, wound healing, energy production and fighting off colds.[65] One advantage of this popular vitamin is that it works together with vitamin E to scavenge free radicals, or stabilize them so they're no longer dangerous. It also helps reactivate used vitamin E so it can continue protecting the body.

In the late 1990's, researchers reported that vitamin C might also help halt the progression of osteoarthritis.[66] This doesn't surprise me in the least. And to further boast about this incredible vitamin, Richard S. Kavner, O.D., who practices optometry in New York City and is former chairman of the Department of Vision Therapy at the State University of New York, says, "Vitamin C helps keep capillaries, the tiniest blood vessels, functioning healthfully. This vitamin nourishes the lens of the eyes."[67] Keep in mind that when you buy vitamin C, make sure it contains bioflavonoids because they help assimilate the nutrient.

VITAMIN E

Vitamin E is another very valuable antioxidant for the body. Before I get into the facts about it, I want to talk about the difference between natural and synthetic vitamin E. As I discussed earlier, always make sure to buy natural vitamins, not synthetic. Natural vitamin E comes in the form of *d-alpha tocopherol* and synthetic vitamin E comes in the form of *dl-alpha tocopherol*. So make sure, before you buy it, to look at the side of the bottle and look for the natural form. Remember, synthetic forms of vitamins are made in a science laboratory and we don't need that in our bodies.

In the eighty years since its discovery, vitamin E has been credited with a wealth of healthy benefits, everything from boosting immunity and fighting cancer to reducing the effects of aging. But "most Americans aren't getting enough of the powerful antioxidant," say Tufts University Researchers.[68] In a statement by Dr. Chris Rosenbloom, associate professor of nutrition at Georgia State University, *"Unlike most vitamins, vitamin E isn't found in sufficient quantity in food to provide the benefits. Research indicates that the amount needed to help the heart is about 400 IU a day, and it's impossible to get doses of 400 IU from food."*[69] Research continues to demonstrate the antioxidant protection of vitamin E from free radical damage, and how it helps stop the beginning of major degenerative diseases. Most studies use supplementation of 100 IU to 400 IU to get positive results.[70] And in a report by Robert Butler, director of the International Longevity Center at Mount Sinai Medical Center in New York, he says that "early in my career I used to tell people to get their vitamins and micronutrients from food. But now I tell my patients to supplement with 400 IU of vitamin E."[71]

Dr. Lawrence J. Machlin is widely recognized as the *world's leading authority* on the science of vitamin E. He is the Director of the Department of Clinical Nutrition of Hoffman-La Roche and is an Adjunct Professor of Nutrition at Cornell University Medical College, and he says, "Vitamin E protects LDL from oxidation, and therefore prevents atherosclerosis (the beginning stage of cardiovascular disease)."[72] Another huge benefit of the vitamin was discovered when researchers from Columbia Presbyterian Medical Center (CPMC) of New York found a person's risk of stroke is reduced by 53 percent if he or she takes a vitamin E supplement each day.[73]

As far as the benefits of vitamin E and our arteries, "it halts the first step in a long chain of reaction that leads to the buildup of plaque in the arteries," explains William Pryor, a vitamin E researcher and director of the Biodynamics Institute at Louisiana State University.[74] And to further this idea through another study, researchers at the University of Texas Southwestern Medical Center observed 24 men ages 25 to 70, ranging from lean to obese, and from healthy to those with apparent heart conditions. One group of men received a three-month supply of soybean oil capsules; the other got identical capsules containing 900 IU of vitamin E. By the end of 12 weeks, the vitamin E level in the blood of those taking vitamin E was 4.4 times higher than in the other group. By the end of six weeks, the LDL or bad cholesterol in the vitamin E group sustained less than half the oxidative damage of those in the other group. Oxidative damage is believed to be responsible for the formation of plaque in arteries.[75]

This information above is a great deal of research on vitamin E that clearly shows its advantage to the body. I highly recommend that you at least take 400 IU daily. But if you are still not convinced, then in the words of Walter Willett, chairman of the Department of Nutrition, Harvard School of Public Health, "For healthy people, there is really virtually no evidence of downsides of vitamin E in the doses commonly used, 200 IU to 400 IU." He takes 400 IU.[76]

9

Other Programs Learned And Explained

During the course of my intense battle with Reiter's Syndrome and Ankylosing Spondylitis, I researched, learned, and performed many programs. Some were unpleasant and complex, while others were quite simple. All proved extremely beneficial and became part of my everyday life. Do not take these programs lightly, because they are of vital importance to help the body get back to its natural state, *disease-free*. Just like in the last chapter, don't worry about trying to do all of these programs at the same time. Rebuilding the body takes time and patience. The best advice I can give is to perform these programs gradually, so you will see the greatest possible results. Below I have explained each one in more depth to make it easier for you to understand and follow if desired. All of the programs below are listed in alphabetical order.

Note: Before using any of these natural programs below, please consult with your doctor. The decision to use them is up to you. After many hours of research, I determined for myself that they were safe and effective. I used them and they all were very beneficial to my success.

CASTOR OIL FLUSH

This was one of the natural programs that was unpleasant, yet very effective. In the morning take 2-3 tablespoons of castor oil and then immediately drink a cup of black coffee. You can add honey or brown sugar if you like for sweetness (try not to use sugar or milk). The unpleasant part of this program will come a few hours later. You will feel your stomach kind of rumbling and then you know what comes next: a trip to the bathroom. Castor oil used to be given to children once a week to make sure they stayed regular. Basically, it's like WD-40 for the gastro-intestinal tract. I know this doesn't sound like much fun, but neither is the pain of arthritis. The goal here is to flush the colon of years of poor eating habits and accumulated waste so that the healing process can begin. I only performed this four or five times during my entire program.

CASTOR OIL HOT PACKS

Castor oil has been used therapeutically for hundreds of years, both internally and externally. Castor oil applied topically has many beneficial effects, and can be used for almost any malady. The castor oil pack is a simple procedure, yet it can produce wonderful results. Some of the effects of the castor oil pack include: stimulating the liver, increasing eliminations, relieving pain, increasing lymphatic circulation, improving gastrointestinal function, increasing relaxation, and reducing inflammation.

You will need the following supplies:

- Castor Oil
- Piece of Wool or Cotton Flannel
- Piece of Plastic or Plastic Bag
- Hot Water Bottle or Heating Pad
- Old Towel

Once you have all the supplies, this is how the hot pack is accomplished. Soak the piece of wool or cotton in the castor oil until it is evenly distributed, but not dripping. Apply this to the joints, liver, kidneys, abdomen, or whatever area you would like to treat. Then apply the piece of plastic over the soaked castor oil. Next place the hot water bottle or heating pad on top of the plastic. And finally place the old towel over the heat to keep everything in place. You will want to leave this on for 45-60 minutes. Personally, I performed this program mainly during the first three months of my program. I used it on my lower back, kidneys, liver, and especially my right toes. I clearly remember after taking the castor oil pack off my right toes, there was less pain and much less stiffness as well.

COLON CLEANSE

The most effective way to cleanse the colon is by way of enemas. This is a program that has been used for centuries, but is rarely talked about or used today due to its sensitive subject matter. This is very unfortunate because the simple enema is one of the least expensive, proven programs in modern medicine. It gently cleanses the colon by flushing out toxins and old waste matter that may cause cancer, colitis, digestive disorders, fatigue, obesity, and much more. *Without proper elimination and bowel function, all other programs, treatments, and supplements will fall short of their potential good.* Plus, it's a much more effective way to clear the colon than taking medications that may or may not work, and are likely to have side effects.

You will need the following supplies:

- Enema Bag
- Organic Coffee
- Vitamin E or K-Y Lubricating Jelly
- Distilled or Purified Water

The procedure is very simple. The first thing you will need to do is fill the enema bag with 12 oz of brewed organic coffee and 20 oz of distilled water, both lukewarm. Then lie on the floor on your right side. This position will enable the water to flow easily into the colon. Next, you will want to place a small amount of the vitamin E at the end of the nozzle for smoother insertion. Once the enema has been administered, the goal is to hold the liquid for ten to fifteen minutes. By that time you should be ready to have a bowel movement to release the liquid and all the toxins contained in it. Please do not underestimate the *enormous* benefit that can be derived from coffee enemas.

DETOXIFYING BATH

This program is one of the more relaxing ones. This bath helps open pores, dissolve and remove toxins, tone and firm tissues, rebalance the skin, and eliminate pain.

You will need the following supplies:

- Epsom Salt (Magnesium Sulfate)
- Baking Soda (Sodium Bicarbonate)
- Ginger in Powder Form

Prepare your bath with hot water (as hot as your body can tolerate). Add 2 cups of Epsom salt, ½ cup of baking soda, and 4 tablespoons of powdered ginger. Soak for 20 minutes, and then rinse off with a cool shower to eliminate any toxins that might be left on your skin.

DMSO OINTMENT RUB

DMSO is easily absorbed through the skin and works well as an anti-inflammatory action that reduces joint and soft tissue pain. It can possibly benefit the following conditions: degenerative arthritis, chronic back pain, muscle pain, tendonitis, bursitis, carpal tunnel syndrome, and general inflammations. Basically, just apply this ointment to any area of the body that needs treatment. You can add other oils like olive oil, castor oil, aloe vera, vitamin E, etc. The action of the DMSO will transport these other oils into the skin and cells where they can be utilized. Just to give you a tip, during the program I would apply the DMSO first, then add some of these other oils, and then put on a shirt or socks to cover the area so it doesn't spread everywhere. I would do this right before bed, and then in the morning I would wake up and the pain and stiffness would be greatly improved.

HOT AND COLD PROGRAM (Hydrotherapy)

This program is very effective, yet most people don't even know it's considered one. It can be done every time you take a shower. It involves alternating between hot and cold water, and it's also known as contrast therapy. Contrast therapies can stimulate the adrenal and endocrine glands, reduce congestion, alleviate inflammation, and activate organ function. Contrast therapies are designed to improve circulation in the digestive areas and the pelvis and to improve the detoxifying capability of the liver. The contrast between hot and cold water increases circulation, promotes detoxification and strengthens the immune system. This helps bring nutrients, oxygen, and immune cells to damaged and stressed tissues. It also helps carry away metabolic waste, inflammatory by-products, and other toxic substances.

The procedure is easy and only takes minutes of your day so there should be no excuses not to do it. While showering, simply apply hot and cold water to the affected areas beginning with hot for three minutes, then cold for thirty to sixty seconds. Repeat three times, and always finish with cold water. Try to make the water temperature as hot and as cold as you can manage to obtain the most benefits. The first time is not easy because when the cold water hits your body, trust me, you will scream and moan. But once you get used to doing this procedure, you will have less pain and stiffness in your joints and feel energized after each shower. It's a caffeine boost without the caffeine.

KIDNEY CLEANSE

The kidneys are the body's filtering system. Keeping them healthy prevents the body from poisoning itself. The kidneys help maintain the delicate balance of body fluids, filter out toxins, and regulate electrolytes and acid content.

You will need the following supplies:

- Juice of 1 Lemon and 1 Lime
- 16 to 32 Ounces of Distilled Water
- ½-1 Teaspoon of Cayenne Pepper
- Honey

In a blender, pour in 16 to 32 ounces of distilled water; add 1 lemon, 1 lime, ½-1 teaspoon of cayenne pepper, and honey to sweeten. Blend it up and drink. On average, I performed this cleanse about twice a week during the first few months, and then once a week thereafter. One of the reasons this drink works so well is because the natural acids from the fruits helps clean the kidneys and urinal tract. Since arthritis is often related to the health of your kidneys, this drink is essential for overcoming the disease.

LIVER/GALL BLADDER FLUSH

The liver is your body's refinery. It plays the principle role in removing from your blood both ingested and internally produced toxic substances. It also makes bile, a yellow-green fluid that is essential for digestion. Bile is stored in your gall bladder, which contracts after eating and discharges bile into your intestines to help digestion. Eating processed and refined foods, eating chemically treated foods, lack of regular exercise, stress, and unhealthy lifestyle choices all combine to alter the chemistry of bile so that it forms solid particles. These solid particles remain in the gall bladder or the base of the liver for many years and become progressively harder, sometimes calcifying into gallstones. When a significant number of solid bile particles accumulate, the free flow of the bladder is diminished, causing progressive stagnation and congestion of the liver. That is the main reason it is so important to keep the liver and gall bladder clean, and to keep the bile free flowing. The liver and gall bladder flush cannot be overemphasized.

You will need the following supplies:

- 8 oz. of Apple Juice (high in malic acid)
- 8 oz. of Distilled Water
- 1-4 Cloves of Garlic
- 1-4 Tablespoons of Extra-virgin Olive Oil
- 1-inch Piece of Fresh Ginger

Start off by pouring the apple juice and water into a blender. Next add 1 clove of garlic and 1 tablespoon of olive oil. Lastly, add the one-inch piece of ginger, and blend it up. You want to start off slowly, and that's why we only used 1 clove of garlic and 1 tablespoon of olive oil. The next time you do the flush, switch to 2 cloves of garlic and 2 tablespoons of olive oil, and keep going until you get to four. Like the kidney cleanse, I would perform this cleanse about twice a week in the beginning and then taper down to once a week. This drink will really help clear your liver and gall bladder of accumulated waste. It was instrumental to helping me gain success in my own program.

SKIN BRUSHING PROGRAM

Skin brushing can be very beneficial because the skin is a primary avenue for detoxification. *In fact, the skin is the largest organ of the body and is also known as the "third kidney"*. It will help improve circulation on the skin and keep the pores of the skin open, encouraging your body's discharge of metabolic wastes. It will also help your skin to look and feel healthier. This program is easy and will only take a few minutes per day.

The first thing you should do is to buy a natural bristle brush (available at health food stores). Make sure it has a long enough handle for those hard–to-reach places. Allow a few minutes before showering so that you can perform the program. Start brushing the skin using circular motions, starting at your feet and working towards your heart. Make sure you brush vigorously and repeat the procedure at least twice. When you are finished brushing you can take a shower, and that's it, you have completed your skin-cleansing program.

VITAMIN C FLUSH

The vitamin C flush is important because it promotes healing of wounds and protects the body from bacterial infection, allergens, and other pollutants. This procedure will make sure that all your body's trillions of cells will be flushed with vitamin C for maximum benefit. *An added benefit for arthritis sufferers is that vitamin C is vital to the production of collagen, which is involved in the building and health of cartilage, joints, skin, and blood vessels.* When buying vitamin C, make sure it includes bioflavonoids since they work synergistically with vitamin C to give it an extra power punch.

Begin the flush first thing in the morning by taking 1 gram (1000 mg) of vitamin C. You will repeat this by taking 1 gram every half hour until you get to the point of slight stomach discomfort or irritation. You might even notice mild diarrhea. This might sound bad, but it's not harmful. In fact, the whole point of the flush is to get to this desired level. Once this level has been established, then you now know your body's vitamin C flush level has been obtained. I determined that my vitamin C flush level is around 18 grams. I still use this program every couple of months or so, and I highly recommend that you do likewise.

10

Arthritis Stopped
My Immune System Wins

"It is the body that is the hero, not science, not antibiotics...not machines or new devices...the task of the physician today is what it has always been, to help the body do what it has learned so well to do on its own during its unending struggles for survival---to heal itself."
---Ronald Glasser, an enlightened M.D.

I have explained the many programs and supplements that I used during my program and the end result is that *I stopped my arthritis!* It took about 16 months of discipline and hard work to become 100% symptom-free. The pain, swelling, and stiffness is completely gone, and even more importantly, my body is no longer attacking itself and causing joint deformities. It was a slow process for me because I was learning the different programs step-by-step. I improved at a rate of about six percent a month. As D.C. Jarvis, M.D., states, "Months are required to cure arthritis- seldom less than three, and sometimes more than eighteen."[1] I believe it could have been faster if I had an outline to follow, but I was treading water the whole way. I didn't know of anyone else that was using natural programs to defeat their arthritis. Looking back at my experience, it certainly was a scary chapter of my life. Hopefully, the path I took can be an outline for you and help guide you to recovery at a much faster rate. *I really be-*

lieve that you can! Imagine: if you are disciplined and can learn to follow these programs, you might improve at 10, 15, or even 25 percent a month. Just think how amazing it would be, if it only takes you four to five months to relieve all your symptoms. It is entirely possible, as long as you never underestimate the power of your immune system to heal itself.

The program I utilized was not easy by any stretch of the imagination. It was the most difficult challenge I have ever faced and accomplished in my life. But at the time, I had no choice. It was either go with a natural program or take medication and most likely end up in a wheelchair for the rest of my life. In fact, at the rate my joints were deforming, I probably would have needed multiple surgeries by now. What choices would you have made, and what choices are you going to make right now if you are dealing with arthritis or a degenerative disease? *It's a matter of self-discipline and personal responsibility versus pain and an unhappy life---I chose to take responsibility for my body, my health, and my life.* I feel that a person really doesn't know what they can handle until they are dropped into a difficult situation. Having a serious health problem forces you to confront that situation to see how you will climb out. Health doesn't just magically appear by taking a drug or a "magic bullet." You have to make a full commitment to be healthy. Every person must accept a certain measure of responsibility for his or her own recovery from disease or disability.[2] The person must understand that the cure is possible only if he is willing to discard completely his former mode of living and accept a new way of life.[3] We all have the strength inside of us to make it through terrible situations like this, as long as we are willing to dig deep to find that strength.

Some people might want to say that I am a "survivor of arthritis." I don't like that expression in the least. I didn't survive arthritis, *I defeated it!* And so can you. I've read numerous books on arthritis that have chapters titled "Hope for the Future," or "The Future Looks Bright." What hope, what future? Those other books don't tell you how to defeat arthritis. They tell you to take medication and "hope" that it doesn't get worse and start deforming your joints. Then, once your joints have deformed past recognition, you will have no other option than to have surgery to replace them. And there's even the chance that you could become bedridden for the rest of your life. *That's not hope, that's a death sentence of pain.*

Many of these books try to impress us by talking about the immune system. They talk about subjects like: DNA, white blood cells, red blood cells, cytokine, TNF-alpha, lymphocytes, phagocytes, leukocytes, etc. If these books and their authors know so much about the immune system, then why is there no cure? The answer is because medications and prescription drugs don't work to help the immune system. The point that I am trying to make is that over the last ten years, I have learned a great deal about the immune system and how to incorporate a better lifestyle into my daily living. It is these lifestyle choices that make the difference between health and disease. In their book, *Preventing and Reversing Arthritis Naturally,* Raquel Martin and Karen Romano, R.N., D.C, state, "Poor lifestyle choices such as smoking and lack of exercise contribute to disease in the body."[4]

In this chapter, I am going to reveal some of the fundamental elements of the body. These are not programs like before, but are basic ways of living. Unfortunately, we don't live in a utopia where everything is perfect and health comes naturally. We have to protect ourselves. How do we do that? By empowering our immune systems to keep us healthy.

IMMUNE SYSTEM

This book is not just about stopping arthritis, but about improving the immune system to stop other degenerative diseases like heart disease, cancer, high blood pressure, high cholesterol, diabetes, etc. I find it painful to watch people automatically reach for the aspirin, cold medicine, flu medicine, or antibiotics every time they feel a little ill. This happens because over the last fifty years, we have been trained by the medical field to do this. Contrary to this popular belief, I have not taken any of these types of drugs over the last ten years. I rarely get sick, because I have empowered my immune system to fight these symptoms, *naturally.* Your body doesn't need these drugs either. The human body is basically the same amongst us all. We all have one liver, one stomach, two kidneys, two eyes, etc. I find it amazing that with the billions of people around the world living in all different kinds of climates, that our bodies' temperature remains the same everywhere. For example, if the temperature in Alaska is 0 degrees outside and in Florida it is 90 degrees outside, our bodies' internal temperature remains at 98.6 degrees. This is not just random luck. This demonstrates that our bodies are all the same and are always trying to maintain homeostasis or internal equilibrium to survive.

Let's look at another car analogy. Imagine if a mechanic found a better way to do a tune-up on a car, but it took a little longer to complete it. The mechanic knew that in the long run, the car would run much more efficient and last longer. It would be very clear to him that he needs to take that extra time to get the job done right. The body is the same way. It may take longer to heal naturally, but once you take the time to do it right, it will be healthier in the long run. With that in mind, D.C. Jarvis, M.D, states, "It is a paradox in our modern world that nearly every machine you can buy is accompanied by a book of instructions telling you how to operate it and make simple adjustments. But the human machine, as old as man himself, has never had any such instructions, *except those which medicine has provided.*"[5] Again, my goal is to try to give you some simple instructions that will help you improve your immune system, not hinder it.

We have to be careful not to let our immune systems trick us. It is extremely important to realize that the various symptoms of disease, such as pain, swelling, stiffness, fever, tiredness, loss of appetite, etc., are not negative phenomena that have to be eliminated and suppressed. Rather, they are positive, constructive symptoms initiated by the body's own healing mechanism in its efforts to restore health.[6] Too often physicians and patients alike assume that a person's symptoms are the disease and that simply treating these symptoms is the best way to cure. Such a treatment is on par with trying to unplug a car's emergency oil light because it is flashing. Although unplugging the bulb is effective in stopping that irritating flashing light, it does nothing to change the reason it is giving its warning.[7] There are many warning signs that our bodies give us: high fever helps white blood cells to be more active; vomiting and diarrhea flushes out toxins; lack of appetite allows the body to focus on cleansing and repair instead of digestion; and fatigue allows the body energy to be shunted away from motion and inward to aid healing.[8] So let's not fall for these tricks, but instead let's acknowledge them, understand them, and let our bodies perform the necessary repairs.

AIR (Oxygen)

Every time we take a deep breath, we are filling the lungs with oxygen so that it can be supplied to the millions of cells in our bodies. Our lungs are a very intricate part of our body and have many important functions. A normal pair of lungs contains about a billion tiny air sacs. Here blood is purified, supplied with oxygen, and sent on its way to the rest of the body. When we breathe out, we exhale carbon dioxide gas and a lot of other wastes.[9] Every twenty-four hours, the amount of carbon dioxide eliminated from your lungs is equal to a lump of charcoal weighing eight ounces.[10] So, a simple rule to remember is that we breathe in oxygen and exhale carbon dioxide. Without this needed oxygen being supplied to our cells, they would die quite rapidly. And just as the goal of live cell analysis is to improve the quality of your blood cells, we should also try to improve the quality and quantity of our oxygen cells. The more oxygen your cells receive, the stronger your immune system will become. But what can we do to improve our oxygen levels?

One of the easiest things you can do to increase the quality of your oxygen intake is to leave you bedroom window open just slightly at night. This will allow fresh air to circulate throughout your room while you are sleeping. Think about it for a minute. Since we all breathe in oxygen and exhale carbon dioxide, if you sleep eight hours a night with your bedroom window shut, you will be breathing in less oxygenated air and more carbon dioxide. I certainly don't want to breathe my "used" air. I can't think of an easier way to get a more refreshing night's sleep than *fresh air*. Give it a try, and after a few days I am confident that you will wake up feeling more energized and more alert than ever before.

Another idea that we can act on to increase our oxygen levels is to perform some type of breathing exercise. There are many different types of breathing exercises that you can select from, but I am only going to describe the one that I utilized. To start this exercise, sit in a comfortable chair with your eyes closed and take a deep breath through your nose to a count of five seconds. Next, hold that same breath for a count of five and then exhale through your mouth while counting to five again. Repeat this same procedure for about five minutes per day. This exercise will help you relax while oxygenating your blood cells at the same time.

With billions of people walking around exhaling carbon dioxide, you would think that sooner or later we would run out of oxygen. Amazingly, in the world we live in all the plants and trees in the world are the exact opposite of us. They use carbon dioxide to survive while giving off oxygen for us to breathe. That is probably why you feel so good after taking a walk in the woods. You have just walked through a fresh "oxygen garden," so to speak. So if plants give off oxygen and use carbon dioxide, it would only make sense to have plenty of houseplants in your home. This is especially true for your bedroom. But not only do plants give off oxygen, they also help detoxify the air. Ordinary houseplants such as the Boston fern, English ivy and spider plants are Mother Nature's pollution-busters, and do a super job of filtering toxins from your home. An example is that a single Boston fern can remove approximately 1,800 micrograms of formaldehyde from the air per hour (an amount in a typical 10 ft. by 10 ft. room). That's sufficient to completely clean the room of pollutants, according to tests by the Environmental Protection Agency.[11] So, providing your home with plenty of houseplants is yet another way to help increase the quantity and quality of the air you breathe.

Earlier, I talked about the benefits of taking vitamins and antioxidants. According to a study in the *American Journal of Respiratory Care and Critical Care Medicine*, a combination of antioxidants was found to protect the lungs of healthy volunteers

Alan Schlines

against ozone, a pollutant found in smog.[12] In the world we live in today, unfortunately, we have to deal with more pollution and smog. That's why it is so important to take extra precautions to keep your body healthy. An easy way of doing this is by taking your vitamins and antioxidants on a daily basis. Sure, a lot of us forget to take them or don't like taking pills, but it basically comes down to discipline and taking responsibility for your own health.

WATER

So far we have talked about the body's first priority, oxygen. Now, let's talk about the body's second most important need, water. It's hard to believe by looking at someone, but our bodies are made up of 70 percent water. *Water is an essential nutrient that is involved in every function of the body.* It helps transport nutrients and waste products in and out of cells. It is necessary for all digestive, absorption, circulatory, and excretory functions, as well as for the utilization of the water-soluble vitamins. It is also needed for the maintenance of proper body temperature. According to Robert Ivker, D.O., and Todd Nelson, N.D., from their book *Arthritis Survival, The Holistic Medical Treatment Program for Osteoarthritis,* "Next to oxygen, water is our most essential nutrient, and drinking enough water to satisfy your body's needs may be the simplest, least expensive self-help measure you can adopt to maintain your good health."[13] And to further this point, in their book *Preventing and Reversing Arthritis Naturally,* Raquel Martin and Karen Romano state, "One of the first things to try when you encounter the pain of arthritis, backaches, headaches, and stomach and intestinal disorders is to nourish the body with generous amounts of water."[14]

But how much water should we be drinking each day? As a general rule, we should all drink at least half of your body weight per day in ounces. That equates to a 200-pound person drinking at least 100 ounces of water per day (keep in mind that a gallon of water is 128 ounces). Why do we need to drink so much water every day? The answer is because your body normally expels about three-quarters of a gallon per day just to function and survive. Personally, I try to drink at least a gallon every day. I start each morning with a 12-ounce glass, and another 12-ounce glass before going to bed. This is to make sure that I start and finish my day on a positive note. I highly recommend that you do the same.

Hopefully, we all agree that water is the key to good health. But let's take it a step further and talk about what type of water to drink. If you are on the list of people out there that are drinking tap water and think that everything is fine, then get ready for what I am about to tell you. *Tap water contains approximately 700 chemicals (129 of which are cited by the Environmental Protection Agency as causing serious health risks)*[15] Some undesirable substances found in tap water are radon, fluoride, arsenic, iron, lead, copper, and other heavy metals. Other contaminants, such as fertilizers, asbestos, cyanides, herbicides, pesticides, and industrial chemicals, may leach into ground water through the soil, or into tap water from the plumbing pipes. Still other substances, including chlorine, carbon, lime, phosphates, soda ash, and aluminum sulfate, are intentionally added to public water supplies to kill bacteria, adjust pH, and eliminate cloudiness, among other things. In addition, tap water can contain biological contaminants, including viruses, bacteria, and parasites.[16] Still further in a comment by Harvey and Marilyn Diamond in their book, *Fit for Life II: Living Health-The Complete Health Program,* "Tap water these days is like a chemical soup. It includes such pollutants as soap, wood pulp, oil, sulfuric acid, copper, arsenic, paint, pesticides, radioactive wastes, agricultural fertilizers, and chemicals from industries to numerous to mention."[17] And if all this wasn't bad enough, a study conducted by the Natural Resources Defense Council found that 18,500 of the nation's water systems (serving some 45 million Americans) violated safe drinking water laws at some point during 1994 or 1995. The council's report blamed contaminated water for some 900,000 illnesses a year, including 100 deaths.[18] So as you can see, if you are drinking tap water then I highly recommend that you stop immediately and switch to a different source, which I will be talking about in just a moment.

You might be a little worried at this point, because you have been drinking tap water for many years and you didn't know it had so many unhealthy ingredients. Well, I have some more bad news for you. It's about another ingredient that has been added to our water sources that is just as bad, if not worse. In fact, whoever had the brilliant idea of putting this ingredient in our water supply obviously wasn't concerned about the long-term health of our country. The ingredient I am referring to is *fluoride.* Are you surprised? Isn't fluoride supposed to be good for us and help protect our teeth? The answer to that is an overwhelming "*no*"! To quote the Diamonds again from their book, *Fit for Life II: Living Health-The Complete Health Program,* "The argument used to convince people that fluoride in our drinking water is beneficial or that it has some positive effect on your health is ludicrous. Go get a dictionary and look up *sodium fluoride*, you will see that by definition it is *a poisonous substance.*"[19] Isn't that great; they have been adding a poisonous substance to our water and can still sleep at night.

There are many problems that fluoride causes in the body. It is known that chronic fluoride use results in numerous health problems, including osteoporosis and osteomalacia, and also *damages teeth*, and leaves them mottled. The salts used to fluoridate our nation's water supply, sodium fluoride and fluorosalicic acid, are industrial byproducts that are never found in nature. They are also notoriously toxic compounds, so much so that they are used in rat poison and insecticides. *The naturally occurring form of fluoride, calcium fluoride, is not toxic—but this form of fluoride is not used to fluoridate water.*[20] It's amazing that they can just add one substance, sodium fluoride, which is very bad for us, but they should have added the correct substance, calcium fluoride. The bottom line is: never drink fluoridated water!

So far we have talked about how water is essential for health, and I have mentioned that tap and fluoridated water isn't good for us. So what type of water should we drink? There are so many different water sources that it can be confusing. There is mineral water, bottled, spring, sparkling, rocky mountain, and many other types. The best type of water that we should be drinking is *distilled water*. Distilled water by definition is water that is vaporized by boiling. The steam rises, leaving behind the bacteria, viruses, chemicals, minerals, and pollutants from the water. The steam is then moved into a condensing chamber, where it is cooled and condensed to become distilled water. Another way to view distilled water is that it's water that has been taken out of the chemicals and pollutants instead of the normal procedure of trying to filter the chemicals and pollutants out of the water. Filtered water will never be as good as distilled water. In fact, distillation is as close as we can get to nature's form of water purification.[21] In the body, this type of water works wonders. *Distilled water acts almost like a magnet in the body. It picks up rejected, discarded, and unusable minerals and, assisted by the blood and lymph, carries them to the lungs and kidneys for elimination from the body. It collects and removes only minerals that have already been rejected or excreted by the cells.*[22] Just remember that distilled water is the preferred source for drinking water.

If for some reason you are not able to find distilled water to drink, there is one exception. The second best type of water to drink is reverse osmosis (RO) water. Reverse osmosis is the finest filtration known (remember, distilled water isn't filtered but vaporized). This process will allow the removal of particles as small as ions from a solution. This water can be obtained from water vending stores, through purchasing a filtration system for your home, or even as bottled water. So if you cannot find distilled water to drink, then reverse osmosis water is the next best thing.

DIGESTION

Quite possibly, digestion might be the missing link to improving your arthritis and other health conditions. Many people in today's world are either too busy to digest their food properly or they just don't realize how import digestion is to maintaining good health. In fact, I feel that many people take digestion for granted. I guess they do this because it's a natural function that will occur regardless of what they eat. So they continue to throw down anything and everything they can get their hands on to satisfy their ever-growing appetites. They expect their stomachs to digest all this food, and to do so without any complaints. Unfortunately, it catches up to them and they begin to experience stomach pains. According to the National Digestive Disease information clearinghouse in Maryland, 60 to 70 million Americans suffer from digestive diseases.[23] This figure doesn't surprise me at all. In fact, I am amazed that this number isn't much higher.

Digestion takes more energy than any other activity that the body performs! It uses more energy than sleeping, breathing, thinking, walking, standing, talking, etc. Living in the fast-paced world that we do, many people are eating fast foods on the go and are never giving their bodies a fighting chance to digest efficiently. With that being said, our goal should be to keep our digestion as quick and efficient as possible. Here are a few things that we can all do to ensure for better digestion.

Habits for Better Digestion:

- Take a Deep Breathe and Relax before you Eat
- Chew Food Slowly
- Eat Sitting Down
- Stay Seated for a few Minutes after each Meal
- Keep Liquids to a Minimum
- Eat Properly Combined Foods
- Only Eat until you are Satisfied, not Full
- Take Food Enzymes with Meals

Try to keep liquids to a minimum while you are eating because they dilute digestive enzymes. This makes digestion more difficult. It amazes me that all these fast food restaurants serve these massive 32-ounce drinks with their meals. How can the stomach even begin to digest this food when it's engulfed in so much liquid? It certainly doesn't make it any easier. Personally, I try to drink 6 ounces or less with my meals. Also, don't eat to the point that you are full, but only eat until you are satisfied.

Another area we need to focus on for proper digestion is the type of foods we are eating. According to Hippocrates, "Man is not nourished by what he swallows, but by what he digests and uses." If everyone is eating too much protein and the wrong kinds of protein, then the digestion process will be very poor, leading to multiple health problems. *Protein is the hardest food to digest and takes the most energy.* The more protein you eat, the less time and energy your body has to complete other tasks, like eliminating toxins. This is an extremely important point for people with arthritis. If the arthritic person is eating too much meat, then the body is spending most of its energy trying to digest it and not spending enough energy on removing toxins and fighting their disease. In his book, *Mysterious Causes and Cures of Illness,* John Matsen, N.D. states, "When the digestion is quickened and made more complete, the body immediately reactivates its healing powers."[24] When we consume excessive amounts of saturated fats (which predominate in red meats) and combine these with altered unsaturated fats (margarines and shortenings) our body can't use them properly, and dumps them somewhere. In rheumatism, that place is the muscles and joints.[25] Our society is so focused on eating enough protein, but when was the last time you read or heard about someone that has a protein deficiency here in the U.S.? Probably never! According to William J. Mayo, founder of the Mayo Clinic, in an address before the American College of Surgeons, "Meat-eating has increased 400 percent in the last 100 years. Cancer of the stomach forms nearly one third of all the cancers of the human body. *If flesh foods are not fully broken up, decomposition results, and active poisons are thrown into an organ not intended for their reception.*"[26] Personally, I don't want active poisons thrown back into my stomach, so I stick with the habits of better digestion to ensure that everything in my body is flowing smoothly.

DIGESTION - MAJOR GATEWAY TO HEALTH

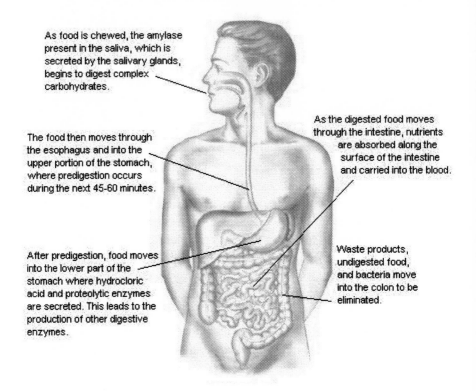

As food is chewed, the amylase present in the saliva, which is secreted by the salivary glands, begins to digest complex carbohydrates.

The food then moves through the esophagus and into the upper portion of the stomach, where predigestion occurs during the next 45-60 minutes.

After predigestion, food moves into the lower part of the stomach where hydrocloric acid and proteolytic enzymes are secreted. This leads to the production of other digestive enzymes.

As the digested food moves through the intestine, nutrients are absorbed along the surface of the intestine and carried into the blood.

Waste products, undigested food, and bacteria move into the colon to be eliminated.

Food Enzymes

As I mentioned earlier in Chapter 8, food enzymes are vital for proper digestion and good health. The use of enzymes in detoxification is important because the body needs an adequate supply of enzymes - not only for digestion, but also for detoxification. Enzymes are best obtained from fresh raw fruits and vegetables, but may be taken daily with meals in the form of a multi-digestive enzyme supplement. Enzymes in our food helps us to digest that food, but many foods today are processed, refined, heated or cooked, radiated and stored, which destroys enzymes and leaves it non-vital. *Foods with enzymes destroyed will have a longer shelf life, but will not give one health when it is eaten.*[27] I want to stress again that enzymes are found in *live foods only*, not the processed foods which are typical of the American diet. And since this is true, it is important that we all take a food enzyme supplement with our meals to help improve digestion.

Why is taking these enzymes so important? *If enzymes are taken with a meal, they help digest protein, carbohydrates, and fat. If taken between meals, they get into the bloodstream where they help do housecleaning.*[28] If digestion fails to liquify meat, spoilage can occur in the intestinal tract - a process called putrefaction. Effects of putrefaction in the gastrointestinal tract are bad breath, foul-odored stool and a general decrease in energy. This is a good reason to supplement the diet with an appropriate digestive enzyme product, both facilitating breakdown of the protein and preventing putrefaction.[29] I cannot over-stress the importance of digestion. Poor digestive activity due to lack of food enzymes can be the direct cause of many health problems. The constant day-to-day irritation of unwanted food particles puts undue stress on the immune system and tires the whole body. This often explains the fatigue that many people experience following a meal.[30]

Food Combining

I'm sure most of you have heard the expression, "you are what you eat." But the idea of what combination of foods to eat, or food combining, might be a completely new concept to you. The basic concept is that you should eat protein and carbohydrates at separate times (please read Harvey and Marilyn Diamonds, *Fit for Life,* for complete details). *Protein and carbohydrates use different types of enzymes to digest food, and mixing them together just confuses the whole digestion process.* Combining certain foods together causes health problems because alkaline juices from the mouth first digest carbohydrates, and then acid juices from the stomach digest proteins. Eating the two foods together results in neutralization of the digestive juices, so that the food takes much longer to digest.[31] And as I mentioned before, the longer food takes to digest, the more energy will be wasted.

The purpose of food combining is to speed up digestion to the point that the intestinal flora has little time to produce new toxins. If digestion can be made so efficient that extra digestive energy is left over, that's what is sent out into the bloodstream to clean out the old accumulated toxins. Thus, it's our surplus digestive energy that does the housecleaning in the body.[32] The main point here is that if you don't digest your food quickly, some micro-organism will digest it for you, making toxins.[33]

Food combining was not easy for me, but I looked at it as a long-term solution. If I could eat properly combined foods at least a few times per week, I felt that was much better than nothing at all. Just keep in mind that every time you eat properly combined foods, you have just provided your body with extra energy to do something else, like helping defeat your arthritis. For example, fruit by itself digests in about thirty minutes. But eat some meat protein with that fruit and now it will slowly move through your intestines along with the meat. It will now take about six to eight hours, in which that fruit will putrefy in your intestines as it digests. That's not a very pleasant thought. Improperly combining foods like this wastes much of your body's energy engaging in digestion. It's much easier on your body to just eat the fruit by itself. The key is to eat properly combined foods at your own pace and remember that a little improvement is better than none.

Properly Combined Foods:

- Fruits by Themselves (1 hour before or 4 hours after other types of food)
- Vegetables by Themselves
- Proteins with Vegetables
- Carbohydrates with Vegetables
- Protein with Protein
- Carbohydrates with Carbohydrates

Ingesting protein with any starchy food, whether it is rice, noodles, or bread, will generate an acidic toxin in the body that produces fermentation, heartburn, and acid indigestion. *This has been known since 1945, when Arthur Cason, M.D., did experiments showing that eating protein and carbohydrates at the same meal retards and even prevents digestion.*[34] The bottom line is that disease begins with faulty digestion long before the first aches and pains, long before there are any symptoms.[35] That's why digestion is so important, and we should never take it for granted. Instead, we should all follow good habits for better digestion.

EXERCISE

Many of you reading this may not like this next subject, but it is one that we cannot overlook. It is the all-important subject of exercise. With up to 60 percent of today's population being overweight, it is time for us to get off the couch and start exercising. In a quote by Deepak Chopra, M.D., author of *Ageless Body Timeless Mind*, "No group is at a higher risk for depression, disease, and early death than people who are completely sedentary, and by now the value of regular exercise for all age groups has been well documented."[36] It doesn't matter if you walk, run, swim, cycle, lift weights, or whatever else you might enjoy; you just have to do it.

I am not going to get specific on how to exercise, as there are numerous books devoted entirely to this subject. But I will say this: there are three main types of exercise that you must do. First there is *cardiovascular*, which is any exercise that increases your breathing and heart rate for extended periods of time to get the blood pumping. Next there is *strength training*, which involves any exercise that you are using muscle resistance to increase your strength. And thirdly, there is *flexibility* exercises like stretching to help posture and blood flow. According to Dr. Jack Soltanoff, a leading chiropractor-nutritionist, "sets of easy stretching motions helps detoxify the system and promote a feeling of youthful flexibility."[37] It is vital that you incorporate each one of these types into your exercise program to reap all the possible benefits. Also, make sure to choose exercises that you enjoy; otherwise, you might not stay with your program very long. As we all get older, the importance of exercising becomes even more important. A number of studies have found that elderly individuals regularly participating in some type of aerobic exercise program have a better quality of life and live longer than individuals who do not regularly exercise.[38]

Besides the obvious benefit of losing fat, why else is exercise so important to us? Simply stated, exercise enhances the transport of oxygen and nutrients into cells. At the same time, exercise enhances the transport of carbon dioxide and waste products from the tissues of the body to the blood stream, and ultimately, to eliminative organs.[39] When we exercise, we detoxify as we perspire through our skin and exhale from our lungs. Some good exercises include jogging or daily brisk walks, yoga stretches, and jumping on a mini-trampoline, which exercises every cell in the body. Exercise slows down the aging process because it stimulates detoxification.[40] Also, exercise is important for stimulating the liver, gallbladder, and intestines, thus helping regular bowel movements, pumping the lymph and vein systems, and raising the body temperature, which in turn aids the immune system.[41] As I stated previously, we need to take control of our own health by empowering our immune systems to become as strong as possible, and one way to accomplish this is through exercise.

Benefits of Exercise:

- Weight Loss
- Increased Muscle Tone
- Increased Flexibility
- Increased Circulation
- Better Stamina
- Detoxifies and Improves the Immune System
- Enhances Overall Health

Let me get more specific on how exercise helps the joints, thus improving the arthritic condition. *Exercising joints causes the cartilage to be compressed, squeezing fluids out like water from a sponge. Then, when resting, the sponge-like cartilage absorbs fluids, taking in nutrients that the cartilage needs to grow, heal and function normally.* In arthritis, this process is interrupted. Without the proper movement of the joint and adequate flow of nutrition, the cartilage begins to shrink. The joint begins to become stiff, degenerate and hurt. When you don't move your body and joints, in effect they become "rusty." Speaking from experience, it's not easy to exercise when your joints hurt. But there is always something you can do. For example, when I was at my lowest point and was unable to walk, I could still manage to climb on to an exercise bike and pedal for about a half an hour. Sure, there was a little pain, but I worked through it and I always felt much better after the exercise. Not only did my joints feel better, but my overall mood and health were at much higher levels as well.

The key to any arthritis exercise program is to increase joint flexibility, muscle strength, and stamina, without putting undue stress on the joints.[42] The best way to do this is to pick an exercise that fits your body and the symptoms you are currently going through. The right kind of exercise can ease your symptoms, help you lose weight, and help take a load off your joints. It also improves immune functioning and enhances your overall health.[43] If you are worried that exercise will make your arthritis worse, don't be. Exercise encourages the flow of cushioning and nourishing fluid into the cartilage. In addition, it strengthens the muscles, tendons, and ligaments that support the joints, which in turn leads to less force being placed on the cartilage during activity. Exercise also increases a joint's range of motion, improves flexibility, and strengthens overall health. Exercise is an excellent "medicine" for arthritis.[44] *The bottom line is that exercise helps to keep joints healthy!*

SLEEP

Experts say that you should be getting at least seven to eight hours of sleep per night. This is usually enough to keep the body healthy. A good night's sleep is important in order to repair muscular micro-trauma that occurs during the day, and also allows our body to make enough endorphins, which decrease pain.[45] *The best fatigue-fighter in the world is a good night's sleep.* If you sleep well, you'll find yourself better able to handle pain, less stressed and depressed, and more energetic.[46] It is especially important for people with autoimmune forms of arthritis to get good sleep, because they are fighting an immune system disease that doesn't just affect the joints, but makes your whole body feel run down and lethargic. Going through my program, there were many days that I just needed to lay down and take a nap. I'm sure many of you out there know exactly what I'm talking about. If you have days that you feel this way, then I highly recommend that you shut your body down and go take a snooze. Sleep is the great restorer—the re-builder.[47]

As I mentioned earlier in this chapter on oxygen, I want to stress again the importance of keeping your bedroom window open slightly while you are sleeping. The fresh air that will circulate throughout the room during the night will really make a difference, and you will wake up feeling more refreshed and ready to face the day. It is an easy thing to do to ensure that you will get a better night's sleep. Also, for those of you out there that have problems falling asleep at night, here is something you can try that is all natural. Try taking some honey. "Honey has long been used in folk medicine as a soporific (causes sleepiness). So if falling asleep or staying asleep is a problem, try taking an ounce or so of honey about half an hour before going to bed. For most people, this is as effective as a sleeping pill, but without the side effect of morning grogginess and the potential for abuse inherent in sleep drugs", says Judith Wurtman, Ph.D., a nutrition researcher at MIT and an expert on the subject. This is just another way to keep the body natural and stay away from polluting the body with unnecessary drugs.

ATTITUDE AND EMOTIONS

When I was diagnosed with incurable arthritis in the prime of my life, my personality changed quite drastically. I became very depressed, scared, and felt hopeless. I stopped talking to most of my friends and had no social life whatsoever. I wanted to find out what was happening and, more importantly, why was this happening to me. I thought to myself, "I was a good person; I didn't deserve to get an incurable disease." That's exactly how I felt at the time. But as I started my programs and learned more about what my body was going through, I realized that it wasn't about deserving to get an incurable disease. Instead, it was about learning how to deal with it. I had to learn how to handle my attitude and emotions.

One of the first things I realized was that if I was having a bad "pain" day and walked around sulking, it only made the pain in my body feel worse. I knew that I had to snap out of it and change my attitude to a positive one. When I did change, I felt much better and the pain seemed so much less. When we wake up each day, we all have an important choice to make. We have the choice of either picking a good attitude or a bad attitude. We can be happy for the things we have in our lives, or walk around sulking all day and making everyone else around us miserable too. This may sound strange, but if I caught myself in a bad mood, I wouldn't focus on the pain of my arthritis. Instead, I would focus on the positive things in my life. For example, I still had two hands and two feet, I still had my vision, and I still had a sharp mind that I could use to focus on my programs and heal myself. I was still alive! Wow, being alive is certainly an important one! *Sometimes we have to stop and realize that there are much worse situations that we could be in, and we should be thankful for what we do have in our lives.*

Here are some ideas that I recommend to help gain a more positive attitude, reduce stress, and have an overall better mental outlook. First, try to eliminate all the negative things in your life. Things like traffic jams, long lines, angry people, and upsetting news on television. Instead, take a different way to work to avoid traffic, shop at less crowded stores, and watch a comedy movie and laugh once in awhile. It's amazing how good laughing is for the body. In fact, research has shown that laughter and other positive emotions rally the body's natural defenses against stress, pain and disease. The study of humor and its effect on the body has a name: it's called Gelotology. A Stanford University professor and well-known Gelotologist has written that, "Besides increasing heart rate and hormone production, laughter moves extra nutrients and oxygen into your body's tissues. This combination, in effect, bathes tensed, stressed, or troubled areas of the body in a healing balm."[48] So go out and rent a bunch of comedy movies and have a great time laughing. I guarantee you that it will take your mind off of your arthritis, and you will feel much better afterwards.

THE AFTERMATH OF MY INCURABLE ARTHRITIS

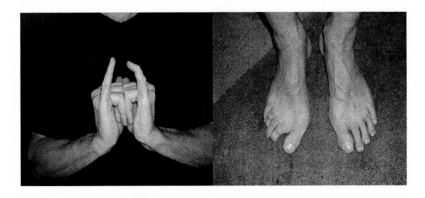

Even though my left pinkie and my right toes became slightly deformed, I can assure you that I have not had any pain or swelling in them for over 10 years. My friends at work and I have nicknamed my pinkie "the claw". Using the natural programs I have outlined, I was able to stop my arthritis before it caused more crippling joint damage.

11

Food Choices:
What's Good, What's Bad

"The doctor of the future will give no medicine but will interest his patients in the case of the human frame in proper diet and in the cause and prevention of disease."
---Thomas Edison

E very day, we all have important decisions that we need to make. One of those decisions is to try to figure out which foods to eat. There are so many food choices that it can become overwhelming. Should we eat fast food? Should we cook our meals at home? Should we buy white bread or wheat bread? Should we drink soda or diet soda? Is it okay to eat fat, and what kind of fat? What types of meat should we buy? Should we buy fat-free foods? What type of oil should we cook with? What foods are healthiest? And to make these decisions even more difficult, if you decide to eat at home then you have the daunting task of going to the store to buy it. Once at the store, it can become very confusing because there are so many products to choose from. You might decide to buy foods that look the most appealing to you. Or you might decide to buy food based on the price. Then again, you might be influenced by advertisements on television or in the newspapers that have caught your attention. Or you might simply be buying the foods that your parents bought out of habit. Whatever your decisions are, in this chapter,

I am going to explain the different food choices based on what I have learned over the last ten years. I will try to make it easy for you and show you what foods your body needs to obtain maximum health and to stay healthy. Eating these healthy foods is the best way to empower your immune system to do its job and keep your body functioning at the highest level possible.

STANDARD AMERICAN DIET (SAD)

If you look back at what you ate today, do you feel that it was healthy food? You might have had coffee and donuts for breakfast, fast food and a soda for lunch, a candy bar for a snack, and a microwaved dinner and a beer for dinner. And to top it off, you probably didn't drink much water. If this is what you ate, then you're probably not alone. You have just eaten what is called the standard American diet (SAD). It's shocking that our country can eat so poorly. Here is another question for you: what is the most important thing that you own? Is it your home? Or maybe it's that expensive car that you have parked in the garage? No, it's not these kinds of things. *The most important thing you own is...your body!* So why are you putting unhealthy food into it?

Let's take a closer look at this standard American diet. Some examples of the things we love to eat are: hamburgers and fries, pizza and beer, hot dogs and apple pie, big steak dinners, coffee and donuts, biscuits and gravy, and fried eggs with ham. To add to all that unhealthy food, let's look at our poor lifestyle choices as well: alcohol, cigarettes, caffeine, eating in your car, on the go, standing up, stressed out, microwaved, eating fast, no exercise, no sleep, burning the candle at both ends. These types of choices are not the ones that will lead to a disease-free body. *After the most extensive study on nutrition ever undertaken by the government, the U.S. Senate Committee on Nutrition and Human Needs concluded in its 1978 report entitled "Diet and Killer Diseases," that the average American diet is responsible for the development of chronic degenerative diseases such as heart disease, arteriosclerosis, cancer, diabetes, stroke, arthritis, etc.*[1] Keep in mind that this study was done in 1978, and it has become much worse since that time. It's no wonder we are becoming un-healthier as a nation. Here are some staggering numbers:

- 1 out of every 2 Americans will develop cancer sometime in their lifetime.
- 1 out of 2 Americans will develop some form of heart disease.
- Breast cancer is a virtual epidemic, affecting 1 out of every 9 women.
- Among men over 50, 1 out of 10 will develop prostate cancer.
- 15 to 20 million Americans over 45 will suffer from osteoporosis, which often leads to severe fractures and even death.
- 14 million Americans suffer from some form of diabetes, which greatly increases their risk of having a heart attack.[2]

It is time to take a step back and look at what we are eating and what type of lifestyle choices we are making. Nearly 60 percent of the population is overweight. Something is terribly wrong with our system, and something needs to be done about it. As I mentioned in the last chapter on digestion, we should all eat until we are satisfied, not until we are so stuffed that we can't get up from the table. Look at our yearly Thanksgiving tradition. Eat until you are so stuffed that you have to loosen your pants, and go take a nap just to recover from the meal. *It amazes me that we can be so oblivious to the fact that what we put in our mouths is directly related to our health.* As Benjamin Franklin said, "A full belly is the mother of all evil."[3] We lead the world in heart disease because we lead the world in consumption of fried foods, animal fats, oils, and sugar. In countries where less fat and sugar are consumed, heart disease is almost unknown. But as soon as our western way of eating gets there, heart disease rates skyrocket.[4] *In fact, many experts believe that changes in the typical American diet could extend the average life expectancy by more than ten years.*[5] So, I'm sorry to say, it shouldn't be a big shock or surprise when all of a sudden you get arthritis, or cancer, or high blood pressure, or any other degenerative disease. Look at what you have been eating for the last 10, 20, or 30 years. This type of nutrition is not what our bodies and our blood cells need to grow new, strong cells that will strengthen the immune system to fight off these types of diseases.

Here is another example of why our society is becoming less healthy every day. I was at the pool a few months ago getting some sun when I heard this 5 or 6-year-old boy whimpering. He was saying, "I want chocolate, chocolate, I want chocolate." It astonished me that this boy was in the pool playing on a nice summer day, and he was crying for chocolate. Then I looked over at the parents, who were notably overweight, and I noticed that they were eating lunch consisting of fast food hamburgers, fries, and those jumbo-size cokes. Of course, the kid was overweight as well. I felt like I was watching the movie "Willy Wonka and the Chocolate Factory" when the little boy, Augustus Gloop, fell into the chocolate river and shot up the tube. I shook my head in disgust. That's what's wrong with the American diet today. The parents are not teaching their kids how to eat right and to select healthy foods. Is it the parent's fault? Not entirely, but I think much of the fault lies with them. I also think that much of the blame is due to another huge factor. That factor is called "advertising."

In the day and age we live in, advertising plays a big role in our lives. Unfortunately, advertising has such an impact on our lives that it can steer us in the wrong direction. If I went and turned on my television, I bet within a half an hour I would see advertisements for fast food, soda, beer, candy, and prescription drugs. If that's not bad enough, we have big Hollywood stars, musicians, and athletes that are endorsing these products to entice us to buy them even more. Do these highly paid stars not care that the products that they endorse are bad for our bodies? Or are they more concerned about how fat their pocketbooks will get for doing these commercials? If they keep endorsing these products, I guess we can say that "the fatter their pocketbooks get, the fatter the people get". I also bet that if I sat down and watched cartoons on Saturday morning that I would see advertisements for some of the worst junk foods possible. Foods like fast food restaurants, sugary cereals, candy, soda etc. After kids watch these ads, they run up to their parents and beg for these products. I am not a parent, but I can only imagine how hard it is to not give in to their kid's demands and buy them these junk foods.

Did you know that advertisers never mention the role that pasteurized and processed foods play in disease, nor the fact that we are routinely ingesting foods containing additives and pre-servatives?[6] Why would advertisers want to mention the facts? Did you also know that over 5000 schools serve fast food in their cafeterias?[7] This is hard for me to swallow, because when I was going to elementary school back in the mid-1970's, there were no fast foods served. In fact, there were no soda or candy machines on the school grounds. We did things the old-fashioned way and brought our lunches to school with us, thanks to our moms. To-day, if you go to a school you will see rows of these machines just waiting for kids to empty their pockets to eat these non-nutritional foods. Again, this just shows you the direction our country is going and why we are becoming less healthy as a na-tion.

Personally, if I reverted back to eating donuts, hamburg-ers, fries, candy, and soda - the standard American diet - then my arthritis would probably come right back. Or this time it might manifest itself as cancer, diabetes, lupus, asthma, etc. *When your immune system is burdened with unhealthy food, it is bound to break down.* To be more specific about arthritis, it is a general observation that the diet of arthritic patients has been deficient in vital nutrients for prolonged periods and loaded with overcooked, canned, frozen, devitalized, and over-refined foods. In addition, the great amount of non-nutritional calories from white sugar and white flour and all the foodless monstrosities made from them makes such a diet even less healthy. This sort of nutritional abuse, combined with other health-destroying factors in the form of overeating, use of alcohol, smoking, coffee, lack of exercise, etc., has caused a general breakdown of our health. It has trig-gered the development of the degenerative process in our joints.[8] I think you can see the point that I am trying to get across. We cannot let our taste buds control our whole bodies. Sure, the stan-dard American diet might taste better, but that's because we have trained our taste buds incorrectly. We need to get back to nature and get back to eating what's natural. We need to re-train our taste buds to enjoy what is good for our bodies, not what you think tastes good. Are you in charge of your body, or are your taste buds controlling your life?

Recommended Dietary Allowances vs. Optimum Dietary Allowances (RDA's vs. ODA's)

If someone recommended that you only take one shower per week, would you listen to them? Probably not. You would survive with only one shower, but people wouldn't want to get too close to you. Instead, you would probably take the *optimum* level of showering, which is daily. It's much healthier for you and you will smell much fresher. Now, let's say you were discussing oil changes for your car, and someone that you just met recommended that you only need to change your oil every 10,000 miles. Being the smart person that you are, you know that your car would probably make it for 10,000-mile oil changes, but you also know that the optimum level for oil changes is every 3,000 miles. Your car will run much better and last much longer. Let's look at one more example, this time using exercise. Let's say you're talking amongst a group of friends, and one of them recommends that, to be healthy, you only need to exercise once per month. Again, you being a smart person, you know that your body will survive by only exercising once a month, but the optimum level of exercise is about three to four times per week. So once again, you make the wise decision and choose the optimum level for a much healthier body. The examples I just described are situations based on *minimum versus optimum*. What do you think is better for you? Of course, the optimum level is better.

Now let's look at the RDAs. It stands for Recommended Dietary Allowance, which is the minimum amount of vitamins and minerals required to prevent a disease from occurring in the general population. *It is not what is required to obtain and main-*

tain optimum health. In order to have vibrant health, you must consider the ODA, or Optimum Dietary Allowance. Here is a chart comparing RDA and ODA:

THE NEXT PAGE CONTAINS THE RDA VS. ODA CHART

COMPOUND	UNITS	RDA ADULT MALES	RDA ADULT FEMALES	ODA OPTIMUM DIETARY ALLOWANCE
Vitamin A	IU	1000	800	5000
Vitamin D	IU	200	200	800
Vitamin E	mg	10	8	400
Vitamin K	mg	80	65	100
Vitamin C	mg	60	60	2000-5000
Folate	mcg	400	400	800
Thiamin(B1)	mg	1.2	1.1	100
Riboflavin (B2)	mg	1.3	1.1	100
Niacin	mg	16	14	100
Pyridoxine (B6)	mg	1.3	1.3	100
Cyanocobalamine (B12)	mcg	2.4	2.4	100
Biotin	mcg	30	30	100
Pantothenic Acid	mg	5	5	100
Choline	mg	550	425	550
Calcium (Ca)	mg	1000	1000	2000
Phosphorus (P)	mg	700	700	700
Iodine (I)	mcg	150	150	225
Iron (Fe)	mg	10	15	30
Magnesium (Mg)	mg	420	320	500
Copper (Cu)	mg	1.5-3	1.5-3	5
Zinc (Zn)	mg	15	12	30
Selenium (Se)	mcg	70	55	200
Chromium (Cr)	mcg	50-200	50-200	200
Molybdenum (Mo)	mcg	75-250	75-250	250
Manganese (Mn)	mg	2-5	2-5	5
Fluoride (F)	mg	4	3	4
Sodium (Na)	mg	500	500	500
Chloride (Cl)	mg	750	750	750
Potassium (K)	mg	2000	2000	2000

As you can see, some of the ODA levels are forty to fifty times higher than the RDA levels. For example, Vitamin E is only set at 10 IU for the RDA, but the ODA is set at 400 IU. Vitamin C is set at 60 mg and the ODA is set at 2000-5000 mg. *These are huge discrepancies!* Personally, I take a good multi-vitamin/mineral along with all of my individual vitamins every day to ensure that my body gets the optimum nutrients that it needs. I want my body to perform at optimum levels. Michael Janson, M.D., in his book *The Vitamin Revolution in Health Care* explains, "Keep in mind that RDAs are not useful in establishing optimum health." He also points out that "while getting the RDAs for certain nutrients will help prevent the corresponding deficiency diseases (i.e., vitamin C for scurvy), these levels do very little to prevent degenerative diseases such as heart disease, arthritis, or cancer."[9] Let me emphasize that last part again, *"RDAs do very little to prevent degenerative diseases."*

FOOD COMPARISONS

At this point you may be extremely confused and don't know where to begin. If you went to the grocery store right now, you would have no idea what to buy or what changes to make in your food selections. That's understandable, due to the fact that our society is accustomed to eating this standard American diet that I mentioned earlier. We all need to get away from SAD and start eating a natural, whole foods diet. The tricky part is knowing which foods to buy. We can start by knowing the differences in food. There are two classes of foods—natural foods and denatured or processed foods. *The natural foods are the only foods that will encourage life, promote strength and endurance, and help to restore lost health.* Denatured or processed foods will always interfere with the normal functions of the body and, sooner or later, cause sickness and disease.[10]

Within my own program, I had to realize that if I ate any of these denatured and processed foods that I would only hurt my chances for recovery from my arthritis. For example, if I had a burger, fries, and a coke then my body would immediately stop the healing process and start using its energy to try to digest and use this unhealthy meal. On the other hand, if I ate a natural meal including foods like brown rice, skinless chicken breast, salad, and herbal tea, then my body would quickly digest and absorb this natural food for its benefit and then continue on with its healing process. It's daily choices like these that make the ultimate difference in your health. In this next section, I will compare certain foods and look at why one is better than the other. You will notice that some of these foods have been debated for years, and I will put a stop to these debates on which products are better for you. I am only going to give you a few examples so you can grasp the basic concept, and then you can make your own comparisons on other foods. The bottom line is that we should eat the foods that will help our bodies become healthier, not the ones that will hurt it in the long run.

Butter vs. Margarine

These two products have been debated for years and I am going to make the winner crystal clear. During the course of this book I have mentioned using common sense and eating natural foods. With that in mind, think about this for a minute. *Butter comes from nature, margarine comes from a science lab; which would you rather have in your body?* Let's look into this even further. If we have butter that is a natural product, then why even create margarine? The reason is that during World War II, butter was hard to come by, so a *synthetic substitute, margarine,* was created to take its place. Margarine is made by turning "pure liquid polyunsaturated oil" into a solid bar of grease. How is the liquid turned to solid? It is hydrogenated—hydrogen gas is bubbled through the oil until it solidifies. It can be made as hard as a block of cement if enough hydrogen is used.[11] Hydrogenated oils in margarine used for cooking break down into dangerous toxins when heated, although butter can be heated for long periods of time without forming toxins.[12]

But what about those commercials on television stating that margarine is "better than butter"? That's just it; it's advertising! You can't believe everything you see on television. You might think you are doing your body good, but it's just the opposite. According to Michael Murray, N.D., as stated in his book *Natural Alternatives to Over-the-Counter and Prescription Drugs*, "Although many Americans assume they are doing their body good by consuming margarine rather than butter and saturated fats, they are actually doing harm."[13] This artificial food should not be used, because it contains ingredients that do not belong in the human diet.[14] *In fact, margarine is absolutely foreign to the human digestive system and compromises your immune system.* Even rodents won't eat it.[15] Besides all the negative effects of margarine, butter actually contains vitamins. Butter contains vitamins A, D, and E, selenium, and iodine. These antioxidants not only protect against disease, but are also required for strong bones and teeth. They also assist in the proper absorption of calcium.[16] So look in your refrigerators, and if you have margarine in there, stop using it immediately. The next time you are out grocery shopping, make it a point to buy butter instead.

Soy Milk vs. Cow Milk

Did you know that we are the only adult species in the world that drinks milk? Do adult cows drink milk? Do adult goats drink milk? Have you ever seen an adult goat drinking cow's milk? It's amazing that as intelligent as humans are, that we are the only ones that find it necessary to drink milk as adults. *Did you also know that milk is the most mucous-forming food on the planet?*[17] In fact, the most serious difficulty with dairy consumption is the formation of mucus in the system. It coats the mucus membranes and forces everything to transpire in a very sluggish fashion.[18] Since my goal is to improve your health, I highly recommend that you eliminate milk from your diet so that your body isn't running in a sluggish fashion.

Did you also know that the calcium in cow's milk is very coarse and hard for the body to digest and utilize? So for all those years you have seen milk commercials on television telling you to "drink milk for calcium and strong bones", this is not entirely true. Again, I stress that you cannot trust all advertising. According to Harvey and Marilyn Diamond in their book, *Fit for Life*, "The calcium in cow's milk is much coarser than in human's milk, and is tied up with casein. Most milk-drinkers and cheese-eaters consume pasteurized, homogenized, or otherwise processed products. This processing degrades the calcium, making it very difficult to utilize."[19] The reason that the calcium is hard to absorb is because the ratio of calcium to phosphorous is out of balance. The phosphorous can combine with calcium in the intestinal tract and prevent absorption. It is also low in magnesium, which is needed for calcium absorption. This can then lead to excess circulating calcium depositing in the joints and arteries, contributing to arthritis and atherosclerosis. So not only is the calcium not used well in the body, it also can cause problems. So when milk companies advertise that "milk does a body good," remember the old saying, "buyer beware."

Here are some other major problems that can occur when drinking cow's milk. Many people are allergic to the protein in cow's milk, which can result in problems such as acne, eczema, constant nasal drip, congested sinuses and asthma. In fact, if you have asthma flare-ups, suspect milk; it is a common culprit in asthma. Going on milk-free diets can cause considerable improvements in some asthmatics.[20] Another problem with milk is that it can be the cause of colic in infants. Recently, Italian scientists got a 71 percent colic cure rate in seventy infants, with an average age of one month, by taking away their cow's milk formulas.[21] With these kinds of results, all the parents out there might want to take note of this. This next one amazes me. It is another case where the American public thinks one way, but it actually does more harm than good. The common sense belief that milk "neutralizes" or buffers stomach acid and helps heal ulcers is a myth. A 1976 landmark study, at the UCLA School of Medicine, proved the point by having normal people and patients with duodenal ulcers drink whole, low fat and nonfat milk. *In all cases, stomach acid levels jumped far above normal levels, and rose highest in ulcer sufferes.*[22] So everyone who has tried drinking milk to help their ulcers, sorry to say, you have just been duped by the "milk myth".

I have explained the negative effects of cow's milk. Now let me talk about the positive effects of soy milk. Soy milk has so many positives that it should be included in everyone's daily diet. Here are some of the main benefits of soy milk.

Benefits of Soy Milk:

- Cholesterol Free
- High in Fiber
- Naturally contains Omega-3 fatty acids and Vitamin E
- Reduces the Risk of Breast and other Cancers
- Great Protein Source
- Not Mucous Forming

Another benefit of soy milk is its *cancer fighting properties*. According to Stephen Barnes, Ph.D., associate professor of pharmacology and biochemistry at the University of Alabama, "Soybeans contain compounds that can manipulate estrogen as well as directly inhibit growth of cancerous cells, theoretically reducing the risk of breast cancer in women of all ages."[23] The soybean has exciting anticancer potential. It possesses at least five known anticancer agents. Soybeans are the richest source of protease inhibitors, which in animals totally block or hinder the development of colon, oral, lung, liver, pancreatic and esophageal cancers.[24] The benefits of drinking soy milk greatly outweigh that of cows milk. I highly recommend that from this point forward, you stop using cow's milk and switch to soy milk instead. I am very confident that you will see a big difference in your overall health.

Wheat vs. White Products (Bread, Flour, Rice, Pasta)

So far, I have given a few examples on how advertising tells us that margarine is "better than butter," and that milk "does a body good." These advertising slogans should be viewed with caution, as I previously explained. Another product that we should be careful with is any product that has the label "enriched" on it. What does that mean? It means that every time a product has the word "enriched" on the package, it has been changed from its natural food state. Let me give you my definition of enriched foods. *Enriched foods are ones that have been unwisely stripped of natural vitamins and minerals, and then enriched with synthetic vitamins and minerals so that it can be sold to the public.* They have to enrich these products, because after they have been stripped, they aren't food. They wouldn't be able to sell these "nothing foods" without this enrichment. Why couldn't they just leave these foods in their natural state? They do it for shelf life, and putting as much money in their pockets as possible.

Let's look at the popular product white rice. What is white rice? White rice is a perfect example of how food processing transforms a nutrient-rich, high fiber food into a nutritional wasteland. In its natural state, rice (which is a brownish color) consists of a husk, bran, and germ. White rice is made by stripping the natural rice of nearly everything that is good, and then throwing in a few vitamins at the end to replace what has been lost. Brown rice, which goes through far less processing, is the whole grain without the outer husk. Because more of the good stuff is left in, brown rice has more vitamins and potassium than does white rice. More importantly, it has nearly twice the amount of fiber, which incidentally is one thing that is sorely lacking in most American diets.[25] Brown rice has had only its husk removed during milling. With the bran intact, it retains more fiber, folacin, iron, riboflavin, potassium, phosphorus, zinc, and trace minerals such as copper and manganese. Moreover, brown rice is the only form of the grain that contains vitamin E.[26] So, when you are cooking foods at home or eating out, try not to eat white rice. Instead, try to only use the natural form, which is brown rice.

Next, let's move on and look at white flour and white bread products. Not only is white flour devoid of its naturally occurring vitamins and minerals, but the less desirable calories are concentrated until they become little more than pure starch and carbohydrate. Why is this abuse of nature's food brought about?

In the case of white flour, shelf life is the main reason. All commercial white flour is processed so that it can be stored for long periods of time. To make this possible, most of the "life" is removed from the whole-wheat berries. Since the oil is removed, it cannot turn rancid. Everything subject to oxidation has been removed.[27] And focusing on white bread, it has a long shelf life because the whole wheat "berry", the part that contains the essential oil and the numerous vitamins and minerals needed by the body to function normally, has been taken out.[28] Once again, these are products that wouldn't be consumable without this enrichment process. Please, just stick with nature and buy whole wheat bread, whole wheat pasta, brown rice, and whole wheat flour products. It is these everyday food choices that will make the difference in your long-term health.

Good Fats vs. Bad Fats

Let's talk about the great fat debate in our country today. Some say it's okay in the diet, and some say that it isn't. I'm going to put an end to the debate right now. There are four main types of fats that we should be concerned with. I have listed them below, with some of their main attributes.

Saturated Fats
Saturated fat is primarily found in high fat cuts of meat, poultry with the skin, whole and 2 percent dairy products, butter, cheese, and tropical oils: coconut, palm, and palm kernel. Eating foods high in saturated fat can cause a person's bad cholesterol (LDL) to rise. The risk of developing certain types of cancer may be associated with a high intake of saturated fat.

Monounsaturated Fats
Monounsaturated fat is found in olive oil, canola oil, peanut oil, and in most nuts and nut butters. This type of fat does not cause cholesterol to increase. When a person substitutes monounsaturated fat for saturated fat, it helps

to lower the bad cholesterol, and protects the good cholesterol (HDL) from going down.

Polyunsaturated Fats
Two major categories of polyunsaturated fats are *Omega-
3* and *Omega-6* fatty acids. Omega-3 fats are extremely
healthful in that they can help a person lower his or her
triglycerides. They also protect against sudden death from
heart attack. Omega-3s are used by the body to produce
hormone-like substances with anti-inflammatory effects.
The best sources of Omega-3s are fatty fish, such as
salmon, sardines, mackerel, herring, and rainbow trout.
Canola oil, walnuts, and flaxseed also contain Omega-3s.

Omega-6 fats are found in oils such as corn, soybean, cottonseed, sunflower, and safflower. *Omega-6 fatty acids
are incorporated into hormone-like substances that promote inflammation.* If one replaces Omega-6 fats with
Omega-3 fats, their total bad and good cholesterol levels
may go down. Omega-3 and Omega-6 fats are not listed
separately on the food label.

Hydrogenated Fats (also know as Trans-Fats)
These are manufactured fats. They occur when hydrogen
is added to a polyunsaturated fat to make it a solid at
room temperature. However, instead of having the quali-
ties of a polyunsaturated fat, it takes on the traits of a
saturated fat. Hydrogenated fats are found in many brands
of margarine, and in vegetable shortening. A clue in determining a less healthy fat is when it is hard at room
temperature; for example, stick margarine has more trans-
fats than softer tub margarine. Now some companies are
making "trans-fat free" margarine products. Beware of
snack items such as crackers, cookies, and chips — many
contain hydrogenated fats because they allow for a longer
shelf life than butter or other fats would. Currently, hydrogenated and trans fats are not listed separately in the

nutrition facts section of the food label. You need to read the ingredient section to find them.

The bottom line is that of these fats listed above, we should focus on consuming monounsaturated fats and omega-3 fats from the polyunsaturated group. That's it, no more debate. The other types of fat are bad for your health and should be avoided as much as possible. *And by all means, avoid the hydrogenated fats, because these are created in a science lab and do not belong in the body.* Below I have included a table showing you the different oils and their amounts of fat. I have highlighted the three that you should be including in your diet: canola, almond, and especially olive oil.

Type of Oil/Fat	% Saturated Fat	% Poly Unsaturated	% Mono Unsaturated
Canola Oil	7	35	58
Almond Oil	8	19	73
Safflower Oil	9	78	13
Sunflower Oil	11	69	20
Corn Oil	13	62	25
Olive Oil	14	12	74
Walnut Oil	14	67	19
Sesame Oil	15	43	42
Margarine	17	37	46
Peanut Oil	18	33	49
Margarine, stick	20	33	47
Wheat germ Oil	20	50	30
Palm Oil	52	10	38
Cocoa Butter	62	3	35
Butter	66	4	30
Butter, whipped	69	3	28
Coconut Oil	92	2	6

I think we all know by now that saturated fats from animal products are bad for us, but another oil that we need to watch out for is omega-6 oil from the polyunsaturated family. Omega-6 excesses worry experts, such as Professor Emeritus Alexander Leaf of the Harvard University Medical School. "When our bodies evolved eons ago, they were nourished by lots of omega-3s and virtually no omega-6s", he notes. "Now, with the invention of processed vegetable oils, the ratio is upside-down in many cultures. Today's fish-deficient diets leave our cells starved of marine oil and overburdened by modern processed oils and meat fats—Big Macs and Mazola oil—foreign to our cells."[29] Of these bad oils, the worst enemies are polyunsaturated fats high in so-called omega-6s, found in abundance in corn oil, safflower oil and sunflower oil, and in the meat of animals fed such fats. "Cut back on vegetable oils with omega-6s, if you suffer from any kind of chronic inflammatory disease," warns Harvard's Dr. George Blackburn. Such pro-inflammatory fats are also a primary reason eating meat can stimulate arthritis.[30] Another reason that people with arthritis need to be careful is because when you consume land-based omega-6 fatty acids from a piece of meat or corn oil, they are apt to be changed into a substance called *arachidonic acid*, which in turn spawns substances that are highly inflammatory or promote blood stickiness and blood vessel restriction. But fat from seafood is radically different and more benign. Its omega-3 fatty acids are apt to be converted into substances that counteract blood platelet clumping, dilate blood vessels and reduce inflammation and cell damage.[31] So we all need to focus on eliminating the omega-6 oils from our diets, and instead eat more omega-3 oils.

Now that I have pointed out the negative effects of omega-6 oils, let me mention the positive effects of this next amazing oil. *It is olive oil.* This is the best oil for us to consume to keep our bodies healthy. Numerous studies have shown that olive oil has a very special effect on blood cholesterol levels; although olive oil may not reduce cholesterol, it does increase the amount of HDL or good cholesterol. High HDL levels are associated with lower rates of heart disease.[32] And to further that concept, a study by researchers at Stanford Medical School of seventy-six middle-aged men with high blood pressure concluded that the amount of monounsaturated fat in three tablespoons of olive oil a day could lower systolic pressure about nine points and diastolic pressure about six points.[33] This is fascinating to me, that eating a fatty oil will not only increase our healthy HDL levels, but it will also help lower our blood pressure. In fact, in Italy, physicians have used olive oil as therapy after heart attacks.[34] So, after looking at the different kinds of fats that are out there, I strongly recommend that you avoid the saturated and omega-6 oils, and include olive oil and omega-3 oils into your eating program.

My Thoughts on the Popular Dr. Atkins Diet

Since I just finished talking about fats, I think it is important to talk about Dr. Atkins and his eating program. This is one of the most shocking diets that I have ever seen. What's even more shocking is that thousands of people have fallen for this nonsense and are taking part in his diet program. Before I begin to talk about his program, let me just tell you that I don't believe in diets. It is a silly concept. If you are eating a wide variety of healthy foods and exercising on a regular basis, then diets are unnecessary. The problem with most Americans is that the foods we are eating are the wrong foods (remember SAD). This is the reason we are becoming more overweight as a nation. Most people don't practice discipline and eat whatever they want, whenever they want, regardless of whether it is healthy food or not. Then when they look in the mirror, "all of a sudden" they need to go on a diet. What we need to do is change our food and lifestyle choices, and then diets will be unnecessary. It takes a great deal of discipline to change our ways, but once you make these changes the rest is easy. The fat will just melt away.

Dr. Atkins diet says to eliminate carbohydrates as much as possible and then your body will burn more fat, thus losing more weight. But by eliminating carbohydrates, you have just eliminated many of the healthy food choices that are available. If you decide to start the Atkins program, then there are no more whole-wheat products allowed, no more fruit, and only certain vegetables are permitted. Some vegetables are considered to have too much starch and you are told to avoid them. Vegetables like potatoes, beets, and carrots are on that list. *I can't believe it: on his diet it's okay to eat sausage, bacon, and hot dogs, but you have to watch out for potatoes, beets, and carrots. And no fruit is permitted...this is absurd!* I ate these vegetables daily to defeat my arthritis, and I didn't eat any of those meats. In fact, I haven't eaten any of those unhealthy types of meats in over ten years.

Consider this for a moment – on the Atkins program, you will be eating much more meat, which also means much more protein and fat in your diet. Meat can cause many problems in the human body if eaten in excess. First of all, there is no fiber in meat. We all know that a high fiber diet is good for us and helps keep us regular. Eating this higher amount of meat, which takes about twice as long to digest as carbohydrates, means that you will have problems staying regular. In fact, you might become impacted on this diet, so be careful. Next, we have to consider the energy factor. A high carbohydrate diet is what provides us with energy. Have you ever heard the expression that athletes use, called a "carbo load"? It's something they do before a big event; load up on complex carbohydrates so that they will have an abundant energy source during the event. I have never heard of a "protein load" for needed energy, have you? So eating high amounts of meat does not provide adequate energy levels. Thirdly, I mentioned that meat takes about twice as long to digest as carbohydrates. So now that you have eaten all this meat, your body is using more energy to digest it. Remember, digestion takes more energy than any other bodily function, so we want our digestion to be as quick as possible. And one more point to focus on: eating high amounts of meat can cause a buildup of uric acid. This uric acid can deposit in your joints and can lead to arthritis. And I think you know by now that my goal here is to defeat arthritis.

So please, don't try to trick your body to burn fat by eliminating the all-important carbohydrate from your diet. Instead, learn to change your eating habits and switch to all natural foods and a healthier lifestyle. What do you think is better for your body? Eating pork, lamb, beef, bacon, ham, fried eggs, and cheese on the Atkins diet program, or foods like lean chicken, fish, turkey, whole wheat, fruits and vegetables on a *non-diet program*? I don't even want you to answer that question, because it is obvious that you should be eating the foods that I have described in this book. I think Dr. Atkins should reconsider what he thinks is healthy and start changing his program immediately, so that all of his followers will at least have a fighting chance at long-term health. In my opinion, if they continue using this type of diet program, then their bodies are at a much greater risk for heart disease, stroke, and cancer.

Salt-Free Seasonings vs. Salt

Earlier in this book I discussed the great importance of increasing your potassium levels and decreasing your salt levels. Your internal cell health depends on having more potassium than sodium. The more sodium in your cells, the more unhealthy they become, and unfortunately, this can lead to disease. In fact, people who use as much salt as they like may excrete nine times as much potassium.[55] This extra potassium loss can lead to an unhealthy future. So why would anyone deliberately increase their salt levels by adding more salt to their food? Do they not care about their health? Or are they more worried about how their food will taste? My opinion is that people are letting their taste buds win the war on health. They care more about the taste of their food than they do the health of their body. This definitely needs to change.

Let me give you some examples of some salt-free seasonings that you can use to replace this destructive sodium. One product that I generously use in my cooking is simply called "all-purpose seasoning, salt-free." The ingredients are as follows: dehydrated onion, parsley, basil, lemon peel, thyme, dehydrated garlic, celery, red bell pepper, citric acid, freeze-dried lemon. It definitely adds more flavor to my cooking than just plain old salt. Another product that I use quite often is called "barbecue seasoning, salt-free". The ingredients in this one are as follows: dried yeast, chili peppers, tomato powder, maple syrup powder, dehydrated onion, paprika, dehydrated garlic, cumin, and mesquite powder. These are just two examples of products that you can use to easily replace salt. This subtle change in your diet can have long-lasting health results.

Mustard (natural) vs. Popular Brand Mustard

Sometimes I wonder what hidden agenda food manufactures are hiding. Mustard is such a simple food, yet many mustard companies add so many unhealthy ingredients to their products. I guess they do it because our society is so infatuated with their taste buds that they keep buying these unhealthy products. Let me give you an example.

> *Mustard's Ingredients (natural):* mustard seeds, vinegar, salt, turmeric and spices.

> *Popular Brand Mustard's Ingredients:* water, sugar, mustard seeds, white distilled vinegar, honey, flour, soybean oil, salt, lemon juice, eggs, garlic, xanthan gum, citric acid, sodium benzoate (preservative), high fructose corn syrup, artificial and natural flavors, paprika, spices, turmeric and annatto, calcium disodium EDTA (retains product freshness).

Why do I need sugar, honey, and high fructose corn syrup in my mustard? That's three different kinds of sweeteners in one product. In fact, why do I need any kind of sugar in my mustard? Why do I need eggs in my mustard? And what is xanthan gum, sodium benzoate, annatto, and calcium disodium EDTA? I'm not making this up. This is straight from the side of the package. What's my point? The point is, and has been throughout this entire book, to stick with natural ingredients that your body needs and can use. Don't eat products that contain unnecessary ingredients that your body has to work extra hard to process. I suggest that you stop buying the popular brand mustard and go buy some natural mustard instead.

Peanut Butter (natural) vs. Popular Brand Peanut Butter

Here we go again with another product that has unnecessary, unhealthy ingredients that your body just doesn't need.

Peanut Butter's Ingredients (natural): peanuts and salt.

Popular Brand Peanut Butter's Ingredients: peanuts, sugar, partially hydrogenated vegetable oils (rapeseed, cottonseed and soybean) to prevent separation, salt.

I really don't think I need sugar and partially hydrogenated vegetable oils in my peanut butter. What do you think? The package says that they put this oil in to prevent separation. How about taking a spoon and mixing it up yourself? That's what I do; it's not a big deal. And I just explained how unhealthy hydrogenated oil is for the body, and that it should be avoided by all means possible. I recommend that everyone should try the natural peanut butter instead, because it tastes just as good. Plus, you get the assurance that you are eating only healthy ingredients.

Fruit Juice (natural) vs. Popular Brand Fruit Juice

By now, I think you can see the idea that I am portraying. Let's look at another example just to clarify my point even further. Below are the ingredients of a frozen concentrated fruit juice.

Fruit Juice Ingredients (natural): concentrated orange, grape, pineapple, lemon, apple, cherry, citric acid, and natural spring water.

Popular Brand Fruit Juice Ingredients: sweeteners (sugar and corn syrup), water, concentrated orange, grapefruit, pineapple, lemon, apple, cherry, malic acid, citric acid, ascorbic acid, natural flavors, carob bean gum, gum arabic and artificial colors (FD&C RED #40 and BLUE #1).

With this product I really have to ask myself, why would I drink something that has two kinds of sweeteners, carob bean gum, gum arabic and red and blue artificial food colorings? I thought fruit juice was supposed to be naturally sweetened by the fruit? And I thought gum was something that you chewed for enjoyment, not eat? Another very important point is that the natural juice is 100% juice and the popular brand juice is only 10% juice - it says so right on the label.

Fruit Jelly (natural) vs. Popular Brand Fruit Jelly

This one is very similar to the fruit juice that I just mentioned.

Fruit Jelly Ingredients (natural): White grape juice concentrate, blueberries, pear juice concentrate, fruit pectin, lemon juice.

Popular Brand Fruit Jelly Ingredients: grape juice, high fructose corn syrup, corn syrup, fruit pectin, citric acid, sodium citrate.

Why do food manufacturers do this to us? I guess they think that our bodies need extra sugar and extra salt to survive. Not only did they add high fructose corn syrup to this product, but they also added corn syrup a second time in the ingredients list. That makes as much sense as drinking a soda and then topping it off with another soda. As the old expression goes, "two wrongs don't make a right." Personally, I will stick with eating the natural products and only put ingredients into my body that will keep it healthy.

LONG-TERM HEALTH

Above, I have just outlined a few products that have many unhealthy ingredients that your body just doesn't need. The reason I did this was to make everyone aware that just because it is a popular brand, or has an appealing package, or your friends down the street eat them, it doesn't mean that it is good for you. They have ingredients that aren't natural and don't belong in the body in the first place. There are many more products out there on the shelves that you should be making the same comparisons with. Why should you? Because eating healthy ingredients all adds up to long-term health.

What does long-term health mean to you? Is it *hoping* that you will be healthy thirty or forty years from now? Is it to eat whatever you want now, and then change your eating habits once you reach fifty? Is it putting your long-term health in the hands of doctors? No, it's none of these things. Long-term health is truly about how you live each and every day that will determine the health of your body in your future. Building a healthy body requires discipline, and making the right food choices on a daily basis. I had a friend say to me once, jokingly of course, "It's okay if I drink too much alcohol today, because in thirty years when my liver is bad, the medical technological advances in liver transplants will be so advanced that getting a liver transplant will be easy". I know he didn't mean this, but I bet there are many people out there with this same attitude. They think that it is okay to indulge and overeat with unhealthy foods, or whatever else they can get their hands on, because the doctors of the future will heal them. There are so many people that don't take responsibility for their own health.

Instead, we need to think of long-term health in the same way as we look at long-term investing. For example, most people are saving money on a monthly basis for their retirement. They are putting money into their 401k's, their IRA accounts, and their savings accounts, etc. They are doing this so that when they reach the age of retirement, they will have a nice lump sum saved for financial security and peace of mind. Well, shouldn't we have health security as well? You might have heard the expression "future value of money." I want to introduce to you a new expression that I call *"future value of health"*. Eating unhealthy food will never give you good future value of health. Only using common sense and eating the right foods for our bodies will give us future value of health. Below, I give many examples of how eating these unhealthy foods all add up to *"future value of bad health"*.

Drinking Sodas Formula

- Drink 2 colas per day
- 2 x 7(days per week) = 14 colas per week
- 14 x 52(weeks per year) = 728 sodas per year
- Each soda has 39 carbohydrate grams of bad sugar
- 1 carbohydrate gram = 4 calories
- 39 x 4 = 156 calories per soda
- 728 x 156 = 113,568 calories per year
- 3500 calories = 1 pound
- 113,568/3500 = *32.4 POUNDS OF UNNECESSARY SUGAR PER YEAR*
- 32.4 x 10 years = *324 POUNDS OF UNNECESSARY SUGAR IN 10 YEARS*

It might seem harmless to drink a couple of sodas per day, but it all adds up in the long run. There is no excuse to put 324 pounds of sugar into your body over the course of ten years for no good reason. And "because it tastes good" is not a good reason to keep drinking them.

Eating Mayonnaise Formula

- Eat 3 sandwiches per week with mayonnaise
- 1 serving of mayonnaise = 11 grams of fat
- 3 x 11 = 33 grams of fat per week
- 33 x 52 = 1716 grams of fat per year

- 1 gram of fat = 9 calories
- 1716 x 9 = 15,444 calories per year
- 3500 calories = 1 pound
- 15444/3500 = *4.4 POUNDS OF UNNECESSARY FAT PER YEAR*
- 4.4 x 10 = *44 POUNDS OF UNNECESSARY FAT IN 10 YEARS*

And you wonder why we are getting more obese as a nation, year after year. I suggest you switch to mustard, *which has no fat*, and you will have much less to worry about, literally.

Eating Candy Bars Formula

- Eat 3 candy bars per week
- 1 candy bar = 14 grams of fat
- 3 x 14 = 42 grams of fat per week
- 42 x 52 = 2184 grams of fat per year
- 2184 x 9 = 19,656 calories per year
- 19,656/3500 = *5.6 POUNDS OF UNNECESSARY FAT PER YEAR*
- 5.6 x 10 = *56 POUNDS OF UNNECESSARY FAT IN 10 YEARS*

How does everybody feel now? You have just put another 56 pounds of unnecessary fat into your bodies. What else can we do to ruin our health? I will show you a few more examples so you can see firsthand.

Eating Fast Food Cheeseburgers Formula

- Eat 3 big cheeseburgers per week
- 1 big cheeseburger = 40 grams of fat
- 3 x 40 = 120 grams of fat per week
- 120 x 52 = 6240 grams of fat per year

- 6240 x 9 = 56,160 calories per year
- 56,160/3500 = *16 POUNDS OF UNNECESSARY FAT PER YEAR*
- 16 x 10 = *160 POUNDS OF UNNECESSARY FAT IN 10 YEARS*

Eating Pepperoni Pizza Formula

- Eat 2 small pepperoni pizzas per week
- 1 pepperoni pizza = 42 grams of fat
- 2 x 42 = 84 grams of fat per week
- 84 x 52 = 4368 grams of fat per year
- 4368 x 9 = 39,312 calories per year
- 39,312/3500 = *11.2 POUNDS OF UNNECESSARY FAT PER YEAR*
- 11.2 x 10 = *112 POUNDS OF UNNECESSARY FAT IN 10 YEARS*

Eating Chocolate Donuts Formula

- Eat 4 chocolate donuts per week
- 1 chocolate donut = 13 grams of fat
- 4 x 13 = 52 grams of fat per week
- 52 x 52 = 2704 grams of fat per year
- 2704 x 9 = 24,336 calories per year
- 24,336/3500 = *6.9 POUNDS OF UNNECESSARY FAT PER YEAR*
- 6.9 x 10 = *69 POUNDS OF UNNECESSARY FAT IN 10 YEARS*

Eating Hot Dogs Formula

- Eat 3 hot dogs per week
- 1 hot dog = 15 grams of fat
- 3 x 15 = 45 grams of fat per week
- 45 x 52 = 2340 grams of fat per year

- 2340 x 9 = 21,060 calories per year
- 21,060/3500 = *6 POUNDS OF UNNECESSARY FAT PER YEAR*
- 6 x 10 = *60 POUNDS OF UNNECESSARY FAT IN 10 YEARS*

Eating French Fries Formula

- Eat 3 large bags of french fries per week
- 1 large bag of french fries = 26 grams of fat
- 3 x 26 = 78 grams of fat per week
- 78 x 52 = 4056 grams of fat per year
- 4056 x 9 = 36,504 calories per year
- 36,504/3500 = *10.4 POUNDS OF UNNECESSARY FAT PER YEAR*
- 10.4 x 10 = *104 POUNDS OF UNNECESSARY FAT IN 10 YEARS*

These examples are the common foods that we eat in our standard American diets. So in a time span of 10 years, we have managed to shovel 605 pounds of fat and 324 pounds of sugar into our bodies. *And that's just with eight different foods!* Imagine if we calculated these formulas on everything we ate. It would be a nightmare! So hopefully you see my point and decide to make a wise investment in your future health value by eating only natural, whole foods today.

THE FOOD COMMANDMENTS[36]

- Thou shalt eat one bowl of whole grain cereal daily.

- Thou shalt eat four cupfuls of vegetables daily- cooked or raw but some of each, preferably half and half.

- Thou shalt eat one cup of whole fruit daily.

- Thou shalt *never* eat margarine, shortening, or hydrogen-ated oils as they depress the immune system and hasten your demise.

- Thou shalt use butter, olive oil, and canola oil as the con-centrated fat in your diet.

- Thou shalt consume a variety of fish, fowl and meats if desired; yogurt, nuts and seeds. Eggs are good food. All of these are in addition to and not in place of the four cup-fuls of vegetables, one cup of fruit and one bowl of cereal daily.

MY 10 WORST FOODS LIST

Many of you will not want to read this list, because these are the foods that you eat on a daily basis. You don't want to face the fact that these foods are all unhealthy. *They are all health de-stroyers.* If you can cut these foods out of your diet, I guarantee that your health will drastically improve. I feel this way because I have faith in the human body and understand that all health be-gins by what you put in your mouth, and these foods don't belong there. So take some pride in your body and stop eating these health-destroying foods. I have put these ten foods in alphabetical order.

1. **Alcohol**
   Alcohol is a poison to the body. It causes metabolic dam-age to every cell in the body and depresses the immune system. The repeated consumption of alcohol inhibits the liver's ability to absorb proteins, fats, and the fat-soluble vitamins (vitamins A, D, E, and K), as well as B-complex vitamins. The toxic effect of alcohol on the liver is very serious. In fact, heavy drinkers are at a greater risk of de-veloping cancers of the mouth, throat, esophagus, and

stomach, probably because alcohol irritates those tissues directly. Heavy drinkers are also more likely to get liver cancer.[37]

2. **Candy**
   Here is a sample of the ingredients that are in a bag of candy: milk chocolate (sugar, chocolate, cocoa butter, skim milk, milkfat, lactose, soy lecithin, salt, artificial flavors), sugar, cornstarch, corn syrup, gum acacia, coloring includes red 40 lake, yellow 6, yellow 5, blue 1 lake, blue 1, blue2, yellow 5 lake, yellow 6 lake, dextrin. It's bad enough that they add milk to candy, but they are also adding milkfat. When was the last time you had an urge for milkfat? Everybody should know by now that these ingredients are not healthy, and will not contribute to a healthier body.

3. **Donuts**
   Here is a sample of the ingredients in a typical donut: enriched bleached flour, water, sugar, partially hydrogenated canola oil, partially hydrogenated soybean oil, glucose, salt, maltodextrin, soy flour, whey, leavening (sodium acid pyrophosphate, sodium bicarbonate, corn starch, mono calcium phosphate) yeast, sodium stearoyl lactylate, mono diglycerides, non fat dry milk, natural and artificial flavor, egg yolks, wheat gluten, honey, agar, carrot oil, cellulose gum, potassium sorbate, citric acid. Some of these ingredients sound like they came right out of a science lab. And once again, they have added sugar and salt. Also, let's not forget about the enriched bleached flour in donuts. *One thing we should never forget is that all foods made with white sugar are the first and foremost destroyers of health.*[38]

4. **Fat Free Foods**
   Here is a sample of the ingredients in a fat free cookie product: sugar, enriched flour, skim milk, corn syrup, fructose, cocoa, glycerin, egg whites, gelatin, chocolate,

soy lecithin, modified food starch, baking soda, corn-starch, salt, potassium sorbate added to preserve fresh-ness, artificial flavor. Just because there is no fat in these types of products doesn't mean they are good for you. What they do to try to trick us is add more sugar to these products. If you look at this product above, you will no-tice that the first ingredient is sugar. *And hopefully, eve-ryone understands that excess sugar in the body just turns to fat.* So when you are buying a fat free food to try to lose weight, it is pointless because the extra sugar will turn into fat anyway and you will be back to square one. Plus, these processed foods are not healthy.

5. **Hydrogenated Fats (Trans-fatty acids)**
These are man-made fats like margarine and shortening that are used in bakery items. Stay away from foods with hydrogenated fats such as cookies, donuts, crackers, and cakes as much as possible. They do nothing for the body other than make it less healthy.

6. **Olestra (Fake Fat)**
Whoever decided to make this product, I really have to question their understanding of the human body. *Humans need fat to survive.* Many vitamins are fat-soluble, and without fat we would not be able to utilize them. Also, we need to provide our bodies with essential fatty acids, which also come from digesting fat. But when we eat olestra, it changes our body's natural flow of digestion. Olestra is formed by chemical combination of sucrose (sugar) with fatty acids, and it has properties similar to those of a naturally occurring fat. But, unlike the natural products, this synthetic substitute provides no calories or saturated fat because it is indigestible: It passes through the digestive tract, but is not absorbed into the body. So in essence, after eating olestra your body will have a diffi-cult time digesting fat, including the healthy fat that our bodies need. Basically, inventing this product was a very bad idea!

7. **Saturated Animal Fats (Bacon, Sausage, Hot Dogs, Red Meat, etc.)**

   Our country is becoming less healthy every year. High cholesterol levels, high blood pressure, heart disease, and strokes are increasing at an alarming rate. What we need to do is stop eating so many saturated animal fats. These types of meat are very hard for the body to digest, and need to be kept to a minimum. Personally, I haven't eaten red meat or pork for over ten years. I stick with lean meats like chicken, fish, and turkey. In a quote by Ernst Schafer, M.D., USDA Human Nutrition Research Center on Aging at Tufts University, "If I had to tell people just one thing to lower their risk of heart disease, it would be to reduce their intake of foods of animal origin, specifically animal fats, and replace those fats with complex carbohydrates—grains, fruits and vegetables."[39] We also know that digesting these types of meat takes much longer than other types of protein. This can eventually lead to colon cancer. In a statement by Dr. Walter Willet, M.D., Harvard Researcher, *"If you step back and look at the data on colon cancer, the optimum amount of red meat you eat should be zero!"*[40]

8. **Smoking**

   I know this isn't a food, but it's so bad for our health that I had to add it to the list. This might be one of mankind's dumbest creations to date. For someone to deliberately put a cigarette into their mouth and smoke it will baffle me for the rest of my life. These things cause cancer and kill hundreds of thousands every year, yet are still legal for sale. I wish someone, like the government, could explain this phenomenon to me. All I can say is, if you don't stop smoking, you will have a very difficult time overcoming disease.

9. Soda and Diet Soda

This drink seems so harmless because it's just a soft drink. But be careful; I mentioned earlier how drinking just two of these a day can lead to long-term sugar abuse. I know it will be hard to stop drinking these, because they are so habit-forming. According to Dr. Royal Lee of the Foundation for Nutritional Research, "Cola is loaded with habit-forming caffeine, so that once the victim becomes accustomed to the stimulant, he cannot get along without it. *There is only one reason for putting caffeine in a soft drink — to make it habit-forming"*[41] But if that isn't bad enough, the ingredients in diet soda are even worse. Methanol, one of the ingredients in aspartame (NutraSweet) is known to be poisonous even when consumed in relatively modest amounts. Disorders caused by toxic levels of methanol include blindness, brain swelling, and inflammation of the pancreas and heart muscle.[42] Woodrow C. Monte, Ph.D., Director of the Food Science and Nutrition Laboratory at Arizona State University, tells us, "When aspartame (NutraSweet) is metabolized, it releases methyl alcohol (wood alcohol), a known toxin that is highly dangerous to humans." He warns us that "once in your cells, methyl alcohol converts to formaldehyde, a cancer-causing agent."[43]

10. White Flour Products (Enriched)

I mentioned this one earlier. These are all the products on the shelves that have been enriched. When you see the *"enriched"* label, put it back on the shelf and look for the whole-wheat products instead. By doing this, you will be giving your body the extra vitamins and minerals it needs to maintain optimum health.

ORGANIC FOODS vs. NON-ORGANIC FOODS

Have you ever thought about where the food comes from that you eat? More specifically, do you ever think about what is sprayed on these foods, and what is put in the soil where they grow? You probably don't think about it at all. You just buy the food at the grocery store, trusting that it is good for you. *Well, keep this in mind: it is common practice to spray foods with toxic chemicals such as pesticides, DDT, dieldrin, dioxin, steroids, antibiotics, and many other poisons.* Spraying with these poisonous substances increases the poisons in the soil, and these poisons are transferred to plants and fruits.[44] It is well documented that the fruits and vegetables we eat contain chemical residues that end up in our bodies. In fact, it has been shown that many of our favorite fruits, such as apples and grapes, do contain high levels of toxic residues from pesticides. These chemicals are being increasingly linked to health problems, especially in children. This poisoned soil will not only help to increase degenerative diseases, but it will also reduce the healing power of the body when brought under special conditions where it functioned favorably previously.[45] What we all need to do is stop and think for a minute about what we are actually putting into our bodies. We all should, according to Dr. D.C. Jarvis from his book *Arthritis and Folk Medicine,* "shun fruits and vegetables sprayed with insecticides and become believers in organic farming."[46]

But why should we switch to organic foods? There are definite nutritional advantages of eating organic vs. non-organic foods. According to a study published in *The Journal of Applied Nutrition* that analyzed the mineral content of organically and conventionally grown apples, potatoes, pears, wheat, and sweet corn over a two-year period, the amount of minerals in organic food compared to conventional food were considerably higher. Specifically, calcium was 63 percent higher; chromium was 78 percent higher; iodine was 73 percent higher; iron was 59 percent higher; magnesium was 138 percent higher; potassium was 125 percent higher; selenium was 390 percent higher; and zinc was 60 percent higher. This is a convincing reason to stick with natural, organic foods. The more our agriculture turns away from natural methods, the more the contents of fruits and vegetables are changed: the sodium content rises, the potassium content diminishes.[47] And when the sodium/potassium balance of our cells leans towards more sodium, that's when disease starts to set in.

But don't organic foods cost more? Yes, they do (this is a problem in itself in which an entire book could be written). But even though natural organic fruits, vegetables and meats are more expensive, it's worth every extra penny to be relatively free of pesticides, chemicals, steroids and antibiotics.[48] Plus, another advantage to eating organic foods is that there are strict regulations for foods labeled "organic." These very detailed regulations assure that any food labeled organic is produced without using most conventional pesticides, petroleum-based fertilizer, sewage sludge-based fertilizers, bio-engineering or ionizing radiation. So as you can see, the benefits of switching to organic are substantial and should be taken very seriously.

COOKING METHODS

Earlier, we looked at different food comparisons to see which foods are better than others. Now, let's look at the best way to prepare these foods by focusing on some different cooking methods. *I made it a point earlier that you should try to eat as much of your food in its natural form, which is raw and uncooked.* Dr. Robert Bell hit the nail on the head when he said, "Man is the only creature upon this Earth that spoils his food before he eats it. Cooked food is dead food. Only living foods can build healthy bodies."[49] But in the world we live in today, it is not very practical or easy to eat all our food uncooked. So when you do cook your foods, hands down, the best ways to cook are either by baking, broiling, roasting, steaming, or grilling them. The golden rule is to never fry or microwave your food.

Cooking Tips:

- Never Fry or Microwave
- Trim All Visible Fat From Meats Before Cooking
- Steam Vegetables Instead of Boiling
- Avoid Cooking at Too-High Temperatures
- Grill or Roast Meat on a Rack so the Fat Drips Away
- Use Olive Oil and Canola Oil for Cooking
- Do Not Use Aluminum Cooking Utensils

This may be the first time that you have heard that microwaving your food is not good for you. The reason is that when you cook by microwaving, you are basically overheating the inside of the food, which in turn causes genetic damage through molecular rearrangement of and destruction to cells. Also, by using this radiation, you are destroying important antioxidants, which are vital to a properly functioning body.[50] And for all you women out there who have just had a child or are expecting, you might want to pay attention to this research that was done. Researchers at Stanford University Medical Center reported that microwaving breast milk just to warm it a little destroyed 98% of its immunoglobulin-A antibodies and 96% of its liposome activity that inhibits bacterial growth, and that the microwave radiation itself may have caused damage to the milk above and beyond the heating.[51] I don't think that anyone wants to lower their baby's immune system by giving them microwaved food. So be careful cooking your foods, and take the time to do it right.

NATURAL HYGIENE PRODUCTS

You might think that I am going a little extreme because of this next topic. But if your goal is to obtain ultimate health and to stop disease, then this topic really does need to be discussed. I keep mentioning that what you put in your body is of vital importance. But what about the things you put on or near your body? Things

161

like soaps, shampoos, deodorant, toothpaste, household cleaning products, and laundry detergent. *These products contain hundreds of chemicals that are not intended to be in contact with the skin.* You can make the same comparisons here that I just did with the foods to see that natural products have the ingredients that were intended for our bodies. Let me give you two comparisons of a natural product versus a popular brand product.

>*Deodorant (natural):* Propylene glycol, water, sodium stearate, aloe leaf juice, witch hazel, lichen extract, glyceryl laurate, coriander fruit oil, chamomile flower.

>*Popular Brand Deodorant:* 19% Aluminum Zirconium Trichlorohydrex, Cyclopentasiloxane, Dimethicone, Tribehenin, Fragrance, C_{18-36} Acid Triglyceride.

>*Shampoo (natural):* Water extracts of nettles, sage, chamomile, kusambi bark, lavender, yarrow, rosemary, wild cherry bark and thyme, sodium Laureth sulfate, Cocamidopropyl betaine, Cocamide DEA, citric acid, methyl and propyl parabens, chloropyllin, fragrance oils.

>*Popular Brand Shampoo:* Water, Ammonium Lauryl Sulfate, Ammonium Laureth Sulfate, Cocamide MEA, PEG-5 Cocamide, Ammonium Chloride, Cocamidopropyl Betanine, Fragrance, Hydroxypropyl Methylcellulose, Tetrasodium EDTA, DMDM Hydantoin, Benzophenone-4, Citric Acid, Dimethicone Copolyol, Methylchloroisothiazolinone, Methylisothiazolinone, D&C Orange No. 4, D&C Red N. 33.

What is C_{18-36} Acid Triglyceride? Do we really need this on our skin? Why do we need Methylchloroisothiazolinone in our hair? It amazes me that these product companies feel that it is necessary to add these unnatural ingredients into their products without thinking about our long-term health. In fact, according to Ted Spence, N.D., Ph.D., "Using chemicalized skin care products is not wise, even though they are less costly. These chemicals may be absorbed into our circulation and provide more 'toxins' for our liver to deal with. We are not made out of cast iron, and even the chemicals in our soaps and shampoos will make a difference with our health."[52] Most people don't see the ill effects of these subtle chemicals, because their liver is able to metabolize them. But, individuals who are environmentally toxic will see a great change in their health when using natural soaps and shampoos. These products might not hurt us today or tomorrow, but what will happen twenty or thirty years down the road?

One of the biggest problems we face today with many of these unnatural products is the fact that they contain aluminum. The popular brand deodorant that I just showed you is 19% aluminum. Why do they put aluminum in deodorant and other products? *Aluminum has been associated with Alzheimer's disease in many research studies.* Early in 1989, the British medical journal *The Lancet* reported conclusions of a British government study: The risk of contracting Alzheimer's disease was 50 percent higher in areas of Great Britain where drinking water contained elevated levels of aluminum.[53] Here are some popular products that contain aluminum: cookware, antacids, buffered aspirin, deodorants, food additives, and shampoos. Do your body a favor and avoid products that contain aluminum. Another thing to watch out for is cooking with aluminum pots and pans. According to a study by the University of Cincinnati Medical Center, using aluminum pots to cook tomatoes doubled the aluminum content of those tomatoes, from 2 milligrams to 4 milligrams per serving.[54] Think about how that can add up if you have been cooking with aluminum pans for many years. So try replacing all your aluminum pots and pans as soon as possible, and also try to eliminate all those toxic household products. Your body will thank you later.

CIGARETTE SMOKING

Why? Why? Why? That is the question that comes to mind. I don't understand why it is legal for sale, why someone would want to slowly kill themselves, and why I have to tolerate breathing it. But the hardest part to swallow is that people who smoke blatantly take their health for granted. There are thousands of people in the world that wake up each morning and are sick with illnesses. They can't get out of bed due to these illnesses, and are in a daily fight for their lives. They don't want to die; they want to live. I was one of these people with an illness many years ago. I woke up every morning in pain and agony, and had to fight to get my health back. But the major tobacco companies, and you smokers, just don't seem to care about health. Every day you poison your body and I guess you think it's funny, hip, or cool. You continue to smoke on these cancer sticks up to the point that you are now sick and fighting for your own life. Now you are one of those thousands of sick people who cannot get out of bed. How does it feel? Stop taking your health for granted, it's a gift from above, not something you just throw away.

I hope you are sitting down, because it is time for some real hard facts about smoking. According to Harvey and Marilyn Diamond in their book, *Fit for Life II: Living Health-The Complete Health Program, "More people die every year because of tobacco than the total number of Americans killed in World War I, World War II, and the Vietnam War combined!"*[55] More American people die *per year* from cigarettes than all three wars combined. So when people talk about how gruesome war is, which I agree it is, maybe we should focus on how gruesome cigarette smoking is. Here are some more cigarette facts.

Facts About Cigarettes:

- A thousand people die of tobacco-related illnesses every day in the United States alone.[56]
- Cigarette smoke contains 4,000 chemical constituents, and more than 40 of them are known to cause cancer in humans.
- Tobacco smoking definitely increases the risk of coronary heart disease and heart attack.[57]
- Smoking causes a serious depletion of vitamin C.[58]

- According to chemists at R.J. Reynolds Tobacco Company, "Cigarette smoke is 10,000 times more concentrated than the automobile pollution at rush hour on a freeway."[59]
- According to K.H. Ginzel, M.D., Professor of Pharmacology and Toxicology at the University of Arkansas, "Smoking-related illness claims in a few days as many victims as cocaine does in a whole year.[60]
- In another statement by Dr. Ginzel, "No drug ever ingested by humans can rival the long-term debilitating effects of tobacco...with the support of stockholders and the sanction of governments, they legally push their lethal merchandise across borders and continents, killing every year two and one-half to three million people worldwide. All things together: *death is in a cigarette*."[61]
- In a bold statement by James Duke, Ph.D., U.S. Department of Agriculture, "Smokers should switch from cancer sticks to carrot sticks and soybeans."[62]

And these things are still legal? What's wrong with this picture? Now that we have looked at some cigarette facts, let's look at the ingredients of these cancer sticks. But first, here is a statement from the Health Secretary that was in the *Los Angeles Times* newspaper back in February 2000. "Tobacco firms have admitted putting 600 secret ingredients and additives in cigarettes, the Health Secretary disclosed....The ingredients include sucrose, cocoa, citric acid and ammonium - which speeds the nicotine 'hit'... (The Health Secretary) said that 'until very recently, nobody knew about any of these ingredients,' adding that he was demanding further information from the tobacco companies so that they could show which brands contained the additives."

Ingredients in Cigarette Smoke:

- *Acetic Acid*
  Used in hair dye and developer.

- *Acetone*
  Used as solvent such as nail polish remover.
- *Arsenic*
  Used in rat poison.
- *Ammonia*
  This is added to cigarettes to add flavor and, some studies suggest, also enhancing the effect of the nicotine in a cigarette.
  "The process of increasing the impact of nicotine by adding ammonia is called 'free-basing', which is similar to the chemical process used to heighten the effects of cocaine. Like cocaine, the nicotine exists in two forms --- acid and base. When ammonia is added, the nicotine converts from acid to base form. The base form can vaporize more easily from the smoke particles into the gas phase, enabling it to deposit directly on the lung tissue and immediately diffuse throughout the body" - Oregon Graduate Institute of Science and Technology.
- *Benzene*
  Used as a solvent in fuel and in industry (dyes, synthetic rubbers etc.). It is known to cause cancer in humans and is particularly associated with leukemia.
- *Cadmium*
  A highly poisonous metal, which is also used to make batteries.
  "Cadmium is more dangerous by inhalation than by ingestion. Repeated or long-term exposure to cadmium, even at relatively low concentrations, may result in kidney damage and an increased risk of cancer of the lung and of the prostate" - US EPA.
- *Carbon Monoxide*
  This is an odorless, colorless poisonous gas that is lethal in large doses. In smaller doses, carbon monoxide causes increased heart rate and shortness of breath. This is because carbon monoxide attaches itself to the red blood cells and so doing hinders the blood's ability to carry oxygen, thus "deactivating" these red blood cells for extended periods of time. In heavy smokers, up to 15% of

the blood may be carrying carbon monoxide, at any given time, instead of oxygen.

- *Formaldehyde*
  Used to preserve dead bodies. In cigarette smoke, this chemical is a known carcinogen and causes respiratory and gastrointestinal problems.
- *Hydrazine*
  Used in jet and rocket fuels.
- *Hydrogen Cyanide*
  Poison in gas chambers.
  "It is among the most toxic chemicals found in tobacco smoke. Short-term exposure can lead to headaches, dizziness, nausea and vomiting" - Health Canada.
- *Lead*
  "Lead is a highly toxic metal. Lead is capable of causing serious damage to the brain, kidneys, nervous system and red blood cells. Children are particularly vulnerable, because lead is more easily absorbed into growing bodies and the tissues of small children are sensitive to its effects. Lead exposure in children can result in delays in physical development, lower IQ levels, shortened attention spans and increased behavioral problems" - US EPA.
- *Mercury*
  "Adults exposed to metallic mercury vapor may develop shakiness, memory loss and kidney disease" - US Department of Health and Human Services.
- *Napthalenes*
  Used in explosives, mothballs, and paint pigments.
- *Nickel*
  Used in the process of electroplating.
- *Nicotine*
  It is this chemical that makes cigarettes as addictive as they are – many studies now suggest that nicotine is as addictive as cocaine and heroin. When you take a drag on a cigarette, the nicotine is absorbed into the blood and eight seconds later it reaches your brain and you get a "hit". This nicotine hit causes other things to happen to

your body, including increased heart rate, increased blood pressure and constriction of blood vessels. The intense "hit" nicotine provides and the fact that it is delivered very quickly to the lungs, the bloodstream and then the brain, makes it extremely addictive. In fact, in between every cigarette, most smokers are actually experiencing mini-withdrawal. Smoking may seem to relieve stress, but it actually contributes to it, and the gentle de-stressed feeling one gets when one smokes a cigarette is actually your body going *"AAAAH! I've got my next nicotine hit, thank you, yes!!!"* Ten cigarettes throughout the day seem to be the minimum required to assuage the nicotine withdrawal symptoms. Nicotine is a damned powerful drug!

- *Phenol*
  Used in disinfectants and plastics.
- *Styrene*
  Found in insulation material.
- *Tar*
  When cigarette smoke is breathed in, it condenses and deposits tar in the lungs. It is the tar that actually transports many of the other chemicals contained in cigarette smoke directly into the body. Tar is a dark, viscous substance that paralyses the cilia (small hairs which protect and clean the lungs) and can also stain teeth and fingernails.
- *Tuluene*
  Embalmer's glue.
- *Vinyl Chloride*
  Ingredient found in garbage bags.

I think the above facts and list of ingredients speaks for itself. If you are trying to defeat your arthritis, another disease, or just try to improve your health, you must stop smoking immediately. The bottom line here, folks, is that every day the newspaper headlines should read in big, bold lettering, *"Cigarettes killed another 1,000 yesterday!!!"* Maybe that would finally get people's attention.

12

Drugs vs. Nature
Which is Safer?

Hippocratic Oath
"I will apply dietetic measures for the benefit of the sick accord-ing to my ability and judgment; I will keep them from harm and injustice. I will give no deadly medicine to any one if asked, nor suggest any such counsel."
---Hippocrates, The Father of Medicine, Written 400 B.C.

You might have a deep-rooted belief that prescription drugs are safer than vitamins and herbs. Maybe you feel this way because you see them advertised on television and at every local drug store that you visit. Or maybe you feel this way because these drugs are recommended and prescribed by our doctors. Well, with that in mind, I am about to reveal to you many well-researched facts that will show just the opposite of this. I will show you an array of statistics that will make it crystal clear that vitamins and herbs are much safer than prescriptions drugs. But before I divulge the facts that prove this point, I want to briefly discuss my opinion on doctors. I want to make sure that everyone understands that I am not biased towards or against doctors in any way. In fact, I believe doctors are amazing people. They go to medical school with the sole purpose of helping oth-ers, which is very admirable. They spend a great deal of money on education and make many sacrifices along the way. Plus, they have to be able to deal with the sight of blood, needles, and all kinds of horrid situations. So, don't get me wrong; I think doctors are lifesavers in certain situations. Let me restate that last phrase: *"in certain situations"*. This is the key concept that we need to understand. The situations that doctors are outstanding in are things like traumas, broken bones, car accident victims, and emergency surgeries. In fact, America is probably the best in the world in this area of expertise.

When it comes to any long-term health issues such as arthritis, cancer, common colds, high blood pressure, high cholesterol, strokes, etc, doctors are trained to prescribe drugs and medications for these illnesses. The doctors haven't been trained to use alternative health methods like vitamins and herbs to treat these long-term issues. *With that being said, doctors have no clue as to the effectiveness of these natural treatments.* It's not the doctors' fault for this lack of knowledge; unfortunately, it is the entire medical system and the type of training that they provide to these doctors (I will discuss this in more detail in the next chapter). The medical system educates their future doctors to kill viruses, germs, and illnesses in the body with drugs. They try to pinpoint where the problem is, and then prescribe a drug that will eliminate the symptom. That is one of the reasons we have so many doctors that specialize in different areas of the body. We have heart specialists, lung specialists, eye, ear and throat doctors, arthritis specialists, and of course many others. I guess they feel that these body parts just go bad by themselves, and need a specialist to take care of the problem. But they seem to have forgotten the simple fact that the body works as a whole, and that each part works synergistically with the others. For example, if your liver is hurting and showing signs of weakness, then you will have other symptoms as well, such as frequent colds, a weakened immune system, and a higher white blood count. These other signs are just as important as your liver hurting, and should never be ignored. So just because all of a sudden your liver has pain, it doesn't mean that you should immediately take a prescription drug and hope that it goes away. In fact, taking this drug will just add a new problem to the original problem. So what does all of this mean? It means that instead of taking a drug to try to alleviate the symptom, we all need to kick our immune systems into high gear and let it do what it wants to do naturally. Your immune system wants to get to the root of the problem and heal itself. Remember what I said earlier: when you wake up every day, your body's number one priority is to survive.

The definition of a doctor, in Latin terms, is *teacher*. They are supposed to "teach" us to be healthier. With that in mind, do you feel that when you leave your doctor's office that you have been taught anything new to improve your health? Let me take it a step further. Forget that I asked if they are teaching you anything "new"; instead, are they teaching you anything at all? Or do they just poke you here and there, and then hand you a prescription that can possible endanger your life? I believe the answer is that they don't teach you anything at all. They just, without even thinking twice, write out that prescription and send you on your merry way.

I want to do something a little different at this point. I would like to challenge all the doctors out there to a simple test. It should be an easy test, since you give these items out all day long and must consider them safe; otherwise, you wouldn't be practicing safe medicine, right? The test goes like this. Let's say you handed out ten prescriptions to ten different patients in a day's time. I want you to go home that night with those same ten prescriptions drugs in your hands, get a big glass of water, and then take them all. Well, are you going to do it...? I doubt it. And even if you did have the courage to take all ten of those drugs, I wonder how well your body will be doing the next month, or next week...or even if you make it until the next day. If you aren't going to take them, then why are you giving them to your patients? I take ten or more vitamins and herbs together on a daily basis. They work together as a team to effectively improve my health. My point is that this entire book is about sharing what I have learned, and to help *"teach"* you to become healthier. Personally, I wouldn't prescribe something that I wouldn't take myself. In fact, I have eaten, swallowed, and performed every program in this book. I practice what I preach. This brings to mind an old biblical proverb that we should never forget: "Physician, heal thyself — then you will be able to heal the sick."

Alan Schlines

FOOD AND DRUG ADMINISTRATION (FDA)

I think it is of the utmost importance that we talk about the FDA for a few minutes. The FDA ensures that the food we eat is safe and wholesome, that the cosmetics we use won't harm us, and that medicines and medical devices are safe and effective. They are authorized by Congress to enforce the Federal Food, Drug, and Cosmetic Act and several other public health laws. The agency monitors the manufacture, import, transport, storage, and sale of $1 trillion worth of goods annually. Further, by definition, the FDA's mission is to promote and protect the public health by helping safe and effective products reach the market in a timely way, and monitor products for continued safety after they are in use. Their work is a blending of law and science aimed at protecting consumers. The FDA is determined to keep these public health protections the same year after year, and to be an effective armor against public health hazards.

Now that I have given you a brief synopsis of what they do, let me get to my point of discussion. *It is a true statement that the FDA regulates both dietary supplements and prescription drugs.* And since their mission is to protect the public health by helping safe and effective products reach the market, you would think that another true statement would be that they would be fair and consistent with both of these products, right? If they regulate one area of products, wouldn't they regulate the other area of products just the same? Don't be so sure about that. The chart below shows the death rates per year in certain categories.

THE AVERAGES OF PER ANNUAL MORTALITY RATES FOR THE YEARS 1981 – 1993[1]

Smoking	400,000
Poor Diet/No Exercise	300,000
Pharmaceutical Drugs	**100,000**
Alcohol-Related Deaths	100,000
Microbial Agents	90,000
Firearms	36,000
Automobiles	23,856
Drug Abuse	20,000
Suicides	19,000
Vitamins	**1**
Commercial Herbs	**0**

-- The National Center for Health Statistics, American Association of Poison Control Centers, Centers for Disease Control and Prevention, the Journal of the American Medical Association, U.S. Consumer Product Safety Commission

Make no mistake about it, that's 100,000 deaths per year from pharmaceutical drugs alone! That's in comparison to only 1 death per year for both vitamins and herbs, *combined.* Does the FDA use different guidelines for these two categories? Are they less stringent on the pharmaceutical drug companies for some reason? They must be, if 100,000 deaths are occurring per year due to these drugs. There is something terrible wrong with this picture. In fact, the Federal Drug Administration themselves publishes annual figures in America of 100,000 to 120,000 deaths per year resulting directly from prescription medications, with a further two million people suffering from moderate to severe side effects.[2] Let me review this again to make sure you understand. If the FDA is in charge of regulating the safety of prescription drugs, and 100,000 deaths per year occur due to these drugs, then the FDA is responsible for 100,000 deaths per year. If we were in algebra class, then this would be a true statement. But there are other factors we need to consider.

Personally, I don't think the blame lies entirely with the FDA. The drug companies are the ones who begin this death toll by making these dangerous drugs. I also believe that the doctors are partially responsible, since they are the ones writing out prescriptions for these drugs. And let's not forget about you, the patient. You have to take some responsibility for these above statistics as well. Nobody is forcing you to take these dangerous drugs. You are the ones who are opening the bottles and popping the pills. Just because your doctor told you to, doesn't mean you have to do it. If I told you to jump off a bridge, are you going to do it? Okay, sorry about the sarcasm. But my point is that we all need to take more responsibility for our own health. I wouldn't be writing this book today, sharing my knowledge with you, if I had merely taken the drugs that my doctor prescribed to me. That's a horrible thought to imagine! Where would I be today if I hadn't gone against the traditional doctors' way of thinking? But back to the FDA - maybe they are being swayed to be less stringent on the drugs that they regulate. Maybe the pharmaceutical companies are giving them some kind of kickbacks. I wonder if money is the reason? I will let you answer that one. Just keep this in mind...according to Jason Theodosakis, M.D., Brenda Adderly, M.H.A., and Barry Fox, P.H.D., in their best selling book *The Arthritis Cure*, "We certainly have a good medical system, but it has traditionally been slow to accept new programs or ideas. This is partially due to the Federal Drug Administration's (FDA) decidedly unfriendly attitude toward the use of vitamins and other supplements for anything other than assuring that you meet your recommended daily nutrition requirements."[3]

SAFETY SATISTICS REVEALED

Have you ever paid close attention to those drug commercials on television? I have, and I find it really odd that at the end of these commercials they have these long warnings that say, "By taking this product you may develop side effects which include heartburn, headaches, stomach pain, diarrhea, dizziness, drowsiness, dehydration, etc., and if you experience these symptoms that you should call your doctor." This doesn't make any sense to me at all. For example, let's say I take an allergy medicine that my doctor prescribed because I get slight allergies from time to time. But now, instead of having allergy symptoms, I have a headache, dizziness, and diarrhea. I think I would rather have allergies than a headache, dizziness, and diarrhea. The doctor who prescribed it just made me feel worse than before I took the medication. *And now I am supposed to call him back so he can give me more drugs to treat these new symptoms? I don't think so!* This just creates a vicious drug loop, where you get caught in taking more drugs to try and deal with your latest symptoms. Maybe instead you should call your doctor back and ask him why the drugs have such bad side effects. Let's look at another chart that overwhelmingly shows dietary supplements are much safer than properly prescribed drugs. Below is a chart that was prepared by Ron Law, an executive director of the New Zealand National Nutritional Foods Association.

STATISTICAL COMPARISON OF FREQUENT CAUSES OF DEATH IN THE U.S.[4]

Vitamins & Herbs	0.0001%
Sports injuries	0.0020%
Lightning	0.0041%
Electrical Accidents	0.038%
Firearms Accidents	0.079%
Poisonings	0.17%
Asthma	0.19%
Home Fires	0.19%
Drowning	0.21%
Murder	0.94%
Suicide	1.41%
Motor Vehicle Accidents	2.20%
Preventable Medical Misadventure	2.40%
Alcohol	4.49%
Properly Prescribed & Used Drugs	5.18%
Smoking	7.19%
Cancer	22.11%
Cardiovascular Disease	47%

This is absolutely alarming, isn't it? The fact is that properly prescribed drugs and preventable medical misadventure have a much greater chance of killing you than simple dietary supplements. This is real information showing real facts. Properly researched, regulated, and prescribed drugs are the fourth most common cause of death - but they are never reported. That's equivalent to a Boeing 747 crashing every day![5] I couldn't imagine waking up every day to the morning paper and reading a headline that says, *"Another 747 Crashes Today With No Survivors"*. I think if this really happened, then we would have multiple investigations of the airline business's procedures to see what is causing so many crashes, and then try to fix it immediately. Yet, it is happening right in front of our own eyes with the drug companies on a daily basis, but nothing is being done about it. Every day, the morning paper could read, *"Prescription drugs kill hundreds more, yet the FDA and our government does nothing about it."* I know that life is sometimes hard to understand, but this is way beyond belief.

Here's another question for you to think about. Doesn't it seem odd that even when the slightest incident occurs involving a vitamin or herb, that it shows up all over the nightly news? It should seem odd to you, because these news stories are incredibly hyped and the incident didn't even result in a death. Let me try using some common sense to figure out this equation. *Drugs kill hundreds daily and nothing is done about it, and a vitamin has a small incident and is spread all over the news.* Sorry, I can't use my common sense on this equation, because it makes no sense at all. It's basically an example of drugs killing so many, and unfortunately little will actually happen to those who marketed and sold these deadly products. But on the other hand, if an individual sold a product that killed hundreds, then that person's business would be destroyed and that person would be thrown in jail for murder. However, since these drugs are made by large pharmaceutical companies, nothing will happen to either them or those involved in the marketing and selling of these products. *Just like tobacco companies, pharmaceutical companies are untouchable.*

But it's not just drugs that are causing these alarming death rates. It's also doctor and hospital mistakes that are contributing to these deaths that we need to watch out for. For example, here is a breakdown of deaths per year from other categories.

- 12,000 deaths - unnecessary surgery
- 7,000 deaths - medication errors in hospitals
- 20,000 deaths - other errors in hospitals
- 80,000 deaths - infections in hospitals
- 106,000 deaths - non-error, negative effects of drugs

These total 225,000 deaths per year from iatrogenic causes! What does the word iatrogenic mean? This term is defined as induced in a patient by a physician's activity, manner, or therapy; it is used especially for complication of treatment.[6] And if these numbers don't shock you, here is another statistic that is beyond belief. A Harvard study reported that over 10,000 people died in one year in New York City hospitals due to doctors' mistakes or malpractice.[7] Now you can see why it is so vital to take responsibility for your own health, and make sure that each day you are making healthy lifestyle choices. It is these daily choices that make the difference in your long-term health. We all need to remember to put our health in our own hands, not the hands of the doctors.

Dangers of NSAIDs and Other Drugs

Below, I have compiled a list of statistics that show the dangers of drugs. This is only the tip of the iceberg compared to what is actually out there in the real world. My goal is to show you the facts so that you are aware of the dangers. Many of these statistics are focused on aspirin and NSAIDs (non steroidal anti-inflammatory drugs) since these are the most common drugs used for arthritis. But I have also listed other drugs to show that it's not just arthritis drugs that cause side effects, but all drugs. So please read this list carefully, because I want to make sure that you fully understand the consequences of taking drugs. And remember that at one time or another, the FDA approved all of these drugs.

- The stomach irritation and blood thinning caused by aspirin can substantially increase one's chance of a fatal hemorrhage.[8]
- Stomach bleeding and immune deficiencies are well-know problems with aspirin.[9]
- A recent study conducted in Europe concluded that, on average, 1 in 1,200 individuals taking a traditional NSAID for at least two months will die from stomach complications, but would not have died had they not been taking medication.[10]
- According to Michael Murray, author of the acclaimed book, *Natural Alternatives to Over-the-Counter and Prescription Drugs*, "More people die each year as a result of peptic ulcers caused by NSAIDs than from cocaine abuse."[11]
- Do not let anyone inject cortisone into your joints. This treatment is suppressive and harms your immunity.[12]
- There are, in fact, more deaths from prescription drugs every year than from murders, auto accidents, and airplane crashes combined.[13]
- Baycol, a widely-prescribed cholesterol-lowering drug, has been pulled off the market after being linked to 32 deaths in the U.S. Fatalities came from a painful muscle disorder called rhabdomyolysis that destroys muscle tissue and causes kidney failure.[14]
- Disadvantages and side effects of anti-inflammatory drugs are that they are more expensive than aspirin and have potential serious side effects, including high blood pressure, fluid retention, easy bruising, kidney and liver abnormalities, gastritis, and stomach and intestinal ulcers.[15]
- It is evident that cortisone is one of those remedies which are so pertinently called "a cure worse than the disease."[16]
- The good intestinal bacteria are killed off along with the bad ones when antibiotics are used. This allows yeast to multiply unchecked.[53]

Alan Schlines

- A study reported in the *Journal of the American Medical Association (JAMA)* on August 22, 2001, was led by two cardiologists, Eric J. Topol, M.D., and Steven E. Nissen, M.D., chairman and vice chairman of cardiovascular medicine at the Cleveland Clinic. According to the Cleveland Clinic data, people taking Celebrex and Vioxx are nearly twice as likely to have a heart attack as people who take aspirin-like drugs to treat arthritis.[18]
- In a recently published report in the *Journal of the American Medical Association*, physicians based in New York and Boston reported on the severe liver damage caused by Voltaren, one of the nation's most frequently prescribed NSAIDs for arthritis. Patients developed hepatitis within four to six weeks of taking the medication, and one died from liver damage several weeks after starting on the drug.[19]
- In the U.S., the chance of hospitalization due to a G.I.(gastro-intestinal) side effect from an NSAID is 1 in 3 people with RA over the entire course of a person's disease.[20]
- It has been estimated that there are more than 75,000 hospitalizations and 7500 deaths each year directly attributable to NSAID use in the U.S.[21]
- Celecoxib is a new and popular NSAID that selectively inhibits cyclooxygenase 2. It is approved for the treatment of both rheumatoid arthritis and osteoarthritis. Recognized adverse reactions include gastrointestinal hemorrhage, hepatitis, abdominal pain, and diarrhea.[22]
- Can the NSAIDs ruin my kidneys? You bet. There is some evidence that NSAIDs can lower the filtering capacity of the kidneys.[23]
- In a shocking national survey, seven out of ten people said they occasionally took antibiotics prescribed by their doctor for a cold or flu—illnesses which these drugs have absolutely no effect on.[24]
- While some studies have shown that NSAIDs can actually slow the progression of RA to some degree in certain people, for most, regrettably, neither aspirin nor any other

NSAIDs can alter the course of RA or prevent joint destruction in the long run.[25]

- Unfortunately, serious gastrointestinal complications among NSAID users usually occur suddenly, with little or no warning. In 1997, more than one hundred thousand people in the U.S. were hospitalized for gastrointestinal problems connected to NSAID use.[26]

- What are some of the side effects of DMARDs? (disease modifying anti-rheumatic drugs) Occasionally, patients may experience visual problems, including change in pigmentation of the retina of the eye or some loss of feeling of the cornea.[27]

- Although arthritic symptoms initially seem to go away when taking NSAIDs, the disease process itself continues. At first the medications deceive you into thinking everything is under control, because the symptoms improve.[28]

- Once cortisone is taken or injected over any appreciable length of time, it will cause such a breakdown of the organs and the functions of the body that often it will be impossible to bring the patient back to a state of health again.[29]

- The excess use of powerful adrenal hormones such as cortisone and its derivatives in the treatment of arthritis is inexcusable. There will be an increased loss of calcium and increased potential of ulcer formation, and the eventual depletion of hydrochloric acid substances from the stomach. Ultimately, cortisone administration will be a disaster. For a short while patients may feel relieved, but in the long run they will be much closer to self-destruction.[30]

- The most common side effects of NSAIDs affect the gastrointestinal (GI) tract. Patients may experience ulcers, bleeding, and perforations. One of the more common findings is simple upset stomach, or dyspepsia. Diarrhea is also common.[31]

- You should not consider over-the-counter nonprescription drugs, even aspirin, safe. Your health is apt to be better if you do not take any of them. Drugs are dangerous; vitamins are safe.[32]

Why are doctors allowed to give us these drugs? *Have they forgotten the Hippocratic Oath of keeping their patients from harm and injustice, and giving them no deadly medicine?* I think doctors need to get back to their roots and stop harming their patients with these deadly drugs. And keep in mind that these are just a fraction of the appalling statistics that are harming people on a daily basis. Let me remind you that over the last ten years, I have taken enormous amounts of vitamins and herbs. On a daily basis, I take anywhere between 20-30 pills that consist of the vitamins and herbs I described in chapters 5, 6, and 8. Is it safe to take this many pills on a daily basis? Yes, of course it is. I am digesting only natural ingredients into my system that my body will be able to recognize and take full advantage of. But keep in mind that you have to use good judgment when taking these supplements, as with anything in life. I am not telling you to go out and take entire bottles; instead, you should follow the directions on the side of the bottle. According to the great Linus Pauling in his book, *How to Live Longer and Feel Better,* "Nobody dies of poisoning by an overdose of vitamins."[33] Personally, I think I will follow the two-time Nobel Prize Laureate's advice and stick with vitamins, not drugs. And to further this idea, in a separate quote by Norman R. Farnsworth, Research Professor of Pharmacognosy and Senior University Scholar University of Illinois at Chicago, "Herbal medicines do not present a major problem with regard to toxicity based on a survey of the scientific literature. In fact, of all classes of substances reported to cause toxicities of sufficient magnitude to be reported in the United States, herbs are the least problematic."[34] So do the right thing and stop taking those toxic, dangerous drugs. Toxic treatments do more harm than good in the long run. The best physician is your own body. We must learn to strengthen its defenses, not weaken them.

13

Health vs. Wealth:
The Money Factor

"It is truly sad times we live in when the amount of money people make in society is more important than making that society healthy."

---Concerned Citizen

After reading the title of this chapter, you might be thinking to yourselves, "If this book is about stopping arthritis, why is he talking about money issues?" The answer to that question is, simply, that since we live in a world dominated by money, it can often cloud a person's judgment and alter their thinking. Many times we make decisions based on how much money we can gain from it, and not based on whether it's actually the right thing to do. For example, the tobacco companies make billions of dollars creating products - cigarettes - that are deadly killers. This product was never intended to be in the human body, yet it is still sold. Should the tobacco companies be making these products? Of course not, but when there are billions of dollars to be made, they are going to do whatever it takes to get it done. Personally, I don't know how the owners, presidents, managers, and employees of these tobacco companies can sleep at night, knowing they are killing so many innocent people on a daily basis. *It's definitely a tragedy!* But even more specifically, I am talking about the entire medical industry, including doctors, pharmaceutical companies, and the medical schools. They all have something in common: a great deal of money to be made.

Let me give you another example. Let's say that when I was first diagnosed with arthritis ten years ago, I decided to stick with the doctor's recommendation of taking medication and hoping for the best. This means that over the last ten years, I would have been paying for office visits, medications, insurance bills, and God only knows what else. And let's say over those ten years, my arthritis became much worse, needing more office visits, more medications, a wheelchair, and even a few surgeries. Wow, that's a lot of money coming out of my pocket and going into the doctors and the medical industry's pockets. In fact, my doctor would have considered me his best friend, because being a long-term patient continues to build his wealth. Now imagine that this same doctor has one hundred patients just like me. That's an incredible amount of money being handed over to the medical industry. Remember, I am not biased towards or against doctors, I am just telling you the truth.

And now let's completely reverse this scenario, and imagine if everyone decided to follow the natural route like I did instead of taking prescription drugs. What happens to the doctors' business? I think you can see the obvious: that doctors who are practicing in long-term health issues such as arthritis, cancer, high cholesterol, high blood pressure, etc. need our business to survive. *And, yes, I did say that they need our business, because to them, it is a business.* If our society is educated in natural methods and programs, then the medical industry would lose billions, if not trillions, of dollars. According to Linus Pauling in his book, *How to Live Longer and Feel Better,* "It is the drug manufacturers and the people involved in the so-called health industry that do not want the American people to learn that they can improve their health and cut down on their medical expenses simply by taking vitamins in the *optimum* amounts."[1] So I pose a question to everyone: are doctors more interested in money or the health of their patients? Maybe if we lived in a society that didn't pay doctors so much, then the health of our country would go up. That brings to mind the words of the great philosopher, Galen, who said, "The doctor must learn to despise money."

Teach Health or Teach Wealth?

Unfortunately, the medical industry is in a catch twenty-two situation. If the medical schools teach the doctors to, in turn, teach us to be healthy, then they would lose enormous amounts of money. But if they continue to do what they are doing now, pushing drugs, then they will continue to make the big bucks. *That is one of the reasons the medical industry wants us to believe that medicine is safe and vitamins are not* (I just proved this point wrong in the last chapter). According to Alan H. Nittler, M.D., in his book, *A New Breed of Doctor*, "I have come to know and believe absolutely that degenerative conditions of the body are usually nutritional in origin." With that being the case, you would think that nutrition would be one of the top priorities on the medical schools class syllabus. *Well, if you think they are teaching nutrition in medical school, then you are in for a big surprise.*

So what are the medical schools teaching doctors about nutrition? Let's take a closer look at the answer to this. Throughout their four years of medical school, plus several years more of residency and possibly further training, many physicians are taught that drugs and surgery are the "best" ways to treat patients. Some medical students take a course in nutrition, but the bulk of them receive absolutely no nutritional/dietary training at all.[2] This is outrageous, that the bulk of medical students receive absolutely *NO NUTRITIONAL/DIETARY TRAINING AT ALL*! So that means that the doctors who are treating you and your loved ones were never taught the benefits of vitamin C, vitamin E, antioxidants, herbs, garlic, glucosamine/chondroitin sulfate, MSM, and a whole host of others that I have described in this book. Sorry, this may seem shocking to you, but I am just presenting the facts. To further back this, research shows that more than 90 percent of today's health problems are either caused or complicated by the way we eat. That's a well known fact. *Yet 102 out of 127 medical schools in the U.S. don't even offer nutritional training for doctors-to-be.*[3] This is truly a sad statement, and we are supposed to trust our bodies and our futures to them. In fact, in 1985 the

President of the American Medical Student Association testified: "Medical education has traditionally focused on the principles of acute episodic health-care delivery, overlooking the concepts and applications of nutrition and preventive medicine."[4] As I mentioned earlier, doctors are great for acute medical emergencies, but when it comes to long-term health issues, they just don't have a clue.

If the above information isn't bad enough, look at what happened to this future doctor. Dr. Gaby, M.D., spent over ten thousand hours of intensive research in the caves of medical libraries. He found myriad reports documenting nutritional therapy as it is linked to the practices of medicine. But in medical school, Dr. Gaby was told to "shut up about that vitamin and mineral research; never mind that it's published in medical journals."[5] This is a perfect illustration of how these medical schools feel about nutrition. It's no wonder orthodox medicine, by its own admission, does not know the cause of arthritis. Since they don't know what causes arthritis, it would then be logical to expect that they don't know what to do or how to go about finding a cure.[6] When your doctor tells you that there is no cure for arthritis, he means that there is no cure for arthritis with a drug or knife. This is because the pharmacological and surgical treatments are virtually the only curative methods accepted and employed by the average orthodox, allopathic medical doctor. And they are 100 percent correct: *There is no cure for arthritis with drug or knife.*[7] Lucky for me, I educated myself about nutrition and natural programs and put that knowledge to use to stop my arthritis.

Since doctors obviously aren't being taught long-term health care in medical school, then are they and their health care associates in it for the money? *A survey of medical students revealed that 83% wanted to become doctors because of the big money they would earn!* The average medical doctor in the United States earns in excess of $300,000 per year if they have their own practice. The top 20% earn over $1 million. Those that have doctors working for them (and heart surgeons) often earn over $3 million per year.[8] That grossly exceeds the average salary in America, which is about $40,000 per year. But hold on, it gets much worse. The pharmaceutical companies are where the real big money is found. In a study done by Levin Associates in 2000, some of the highest earnings are in pharmaceuticals, where the average salary was $781,256 and the median was $731,271.[9] That is an amazing amount of money to earn in one year, just to sell drugs. In my opinion I think a good term for them is "legal drug pushers." This reminds me of an article I read in June 2002 in the business section of the *Orange County Register*. It listed the top 100 highest-paid executives. In the top 100 were 5 from the same pharmaceutical company. It's a well-known company that has commercials on television for allergy sufferers (I won't mention the name of the drug). Four of those five executives made over $3.4 million. That's right, I'll say it again: $3.4 million in one year. And the highest paid employee of that company made an enormous $12.3 million. In my opinion, this is completely ridiculous. These executives are paid huge sums of money for a drug that is supposed to stop allergies. Instead, how about taking 3-4 grams of vitamin C per day, some vitamin B-complex, and some antioxidant supplements, cut back on dairy products, and of course drink more water. I am confident that you will have better results, without the side effects of taking these types of drugs. Hopefully, if people discover that natural programs work, then these executives will lose their high-paying salaries. Let's not forget about the tobacco companies. The tobacco companies pull in more than $20 billion a year selling a product that causes incalculable pain, suffering, anguish, and death.[10]

Here is a quote from Dr. Marcus Laux, a leading Naturopathic Doctor: "The medical establishment has spent the last 50 years trying to suppress vitamins, minerals and herbs in order to convince the public that expensive, toxic drugs and dangerous surgery are the only possible remedies. The reason for this is since *natural medicines from plant sources cannot be patented*, drug companies, who can mark up their patented pills up to 3000 percent are not interested. And they obviously don't want you to be interested in them either. That's why they continue to discredit natural medicines in any way they can, even if it means spreading misinformation."[11] The key point to remember here is the patent process. *Chemical World*, a business magazine that services the pharmaceutical and drug industry as well as other chemical users, recently reported, "The drug business is one of the most profitable industries in the world. The reason is that the federal government gives the drug companies a monopoly on a newly patented drug for 17 years, and they can charge any price they wish. No one can copy that drug or create a generic for 17 years."[12] And according to Jason Theodosakis, M.D., M.S., M.P.H., Brenda Adderly, M.H.A., and Barry Fox, Ph.D., in their book *The Arthritis Cure*, "You see, drug companies like to put their money into products they can patent, like drugs. The patent protects their product, allowing them to corner the market and make a lot of money. Since they can't patent supplements, they don't want to work with them. They don't invest money to study the supplements, and they don't flood doctors' offices with free samples or information about the supplements (as they do with their drugs)."[13] *So when it comes to making a decision about who benefits from drugs, just remember that most drugs are not developed to enrich your life, but to enrich those who make, prescribe and sell them.*[14]

Shocking Health Statistics

- Recent estimates suggest that each year, more than 1 million patients are injured while in the hospital, and approximately 180,000 die because of these injuries. Furthermore, drug-related morbidity and mortality are common and are estimated to cost more than $136 billion a year.[15]
- Drug costs are higher in the U.S. than anywhere else in the world.[16]
- Often it takes 10 years from creation through testing until a drug comes to market. Drug companies claim the cost ranges from $50 million to $250 million per drug. Let's say a drug company spent $200 million, and it discovered some problems with the drug. A $200 million investment is a mighty big incentive to downplay the problems. *Time Magazine* quoted Robert Temple, chief of the FDA's Of-

fice of Drug Evaluation, as saying, "They definitely have rose-colored glasses!"[17]

- Bypass surgery—a $10 million-a-day industry—manages to reduce the population by some 28,000 patients annually. Angioplasty is a $4 billion business and sends nearly 9,000 patients a year to an early grave.[18]

- The Institute of Medicine is part of the National Academy of Sciences, a private organization chartered by Congress to advise the government on scientific matter. In one of their reports, it was stated that "the total cost of medical mistakes, lost income and production, cost of disability and health care, totals $17 to 29 billion a year."[19]

- In the United States alone, over $400 million is spent annually on laxatives. This year an estimated 130,000 new cases of colon and rectal cancer will be diagnosed, making it the fourth most common form of cancer in Americans. Of this population, approximately 44% will die as a result of the disease.[20]

- Total sales of RA therapies in 1999 worldwide were almost $1.5 billion. With the advent of new NSAIDs, the adoption of unique biologics, and the promise of others to follow, estimates of $6.6 billion by 2009, with $4.5 billion of that in biologics sales alone seems realistic.[21]

- Sandoz Pharmaceuticals found a simple way to double its profits: water down the medicine by 50 percent, put it in the same size bottle and charge the same price! According to *U.S News & World Report*, attorney generals in 34 states accused Sandoz of doing exactly that with their Triaminic Cold and Cough medicine for children. And they had the gall to call it "New and Improved".[22]

- According to the World Health Association, 60 percent of doctors today prescribe antibiotics for the common cold, even though they know that antibiotics do not protect against viral infections.[23]

Alan Schlines

Are We the Healthiest Country?

Living in the United States is an incredible experience, and every day I feel fortunate that I have that opportunity. But with that being said, there is a topic we need to focus on in much greater detail. That topic is the health of our country. *The United States spends more money on health care than any country in the world.* For 1994, the projection is that the total will exceed one trillion dollars.[24] With that exuberant amount of money being spent (and this statistic is from almost ten years ago), it would then be a logical conclusion to say that we should be the healthiest country in the world. Isn't that how things usually work - the most money means the best, right? Amazingly, we are not even close. *Of 13 countries in a recent comparison, the United States ranks an average of 12th out of 14 for 16 available health indicators.*[25] This poor performance of the U.S. was further confirmed by a World Health Organization study, which used different data and ranked the United States as 15th among 25 industrialized countries.[26]. With that much money being spent, we should definitely be ranked first, not 15th. And to add even more bad news, the U.S. is ranked 16th in terms of life expectancy, and there are more people in nursing homes in this country than anywhere else in the world.[27] What about medical technology? That's important to consider when looking at the statistics, right? Lack of technology is certainly not a contributing factor to the U.S.'s low ranking. Among 29 countries, the U.S. is second only to Japan in the availability of magnetic resonance imaging units and computed tomography scanners per million populations. However, Japan ranks highest in health, whereas the U.S. ranks among the lowest.[28] In the words of John Matsen, N.D., from his book *Mysterious Causes and Cures of Illness,* "Education, not expensive technology, is the key to health."[29]

Speaking of bad news, let's look at the health of our country from a different perspective. The leading causes of death in the United States in 1999 was heart disease at 769,353 deaths, followed by cancer with 476,927 deaths, and cerebrovascular disease (strokes) with 149,835 deaths.[30] These numbers seem surprisingly high – and hard to believe, since we spend the most money on health care. Yet you can walk down any street in the U.S. and see that over half of the population is overweight, hospitals are overflowing, and patients are backed up waiting for surgery.[31] I guess it is like my math teacher used to tell me: "Statistics don't lie," so unfortunately we have to trust them. Personally, I feel that much of this health care money is spent on unnecessary surgeries; surgeries that can be avoided with better food choices and better lifestyle choices, as I mentioned in my earlier chapters. In 1977 there were 50,000 bypass heart surgeries, and in 1986 there were over 200,000 of them.[32] These numbers are growing at a horrific rate, and today that would put us up around 500,000 heart surgeries per year. Are that many surgeries really necessary? No, they are not. *Per capita, Americans have twice as many bypass surgeries as Canadians and five times as many as the people of France. Yet 20 percent more people in the United States die of heart disease than in Canada per capita.*[33] These numbers suggest that the surgeries aren't helping very much. So, what would happen if doctors went on strike and stopped performing these surgeries and other procedures? The last time doctors in Los Angeles took to the picket lines to protest the high cost of malpractice insurance, the result was an 18 percent drop in the death rate during this period. In Bogota, Columbia, that same year, striking doctors refused to handle all but emergency cases, and the death rate dropped 35 percent.[34] As I mentioned before, doctors are great for emergency care, but not long-term health issues. Long-term health issues such as heart disease, high blood pressure, and arthritis can all be easily avoided by empowering your immune system to overcome these types of diseases.

Since this book is focused on arthritis, let me get more specific with the health of our country in regards to this topic. Remember, we spend the most money on health care, so a little thing like arthritis shouldn't be a big deal, right? I'm sorry to inform you, but arthritis is a huge problem in this country. *Arthritis is the leading cause of disability in the U.S.* In 1998, arthritis and other rheumatic conditions affected 43 million people - a number that is expected to climb to 60 million by 2020 as the "baby boom" generation ages. That's almost 20 percent of the population.[35]

**Leading Causes of Disability Among Persons
Aged 15 Years and Older**
United States, 1991–1992

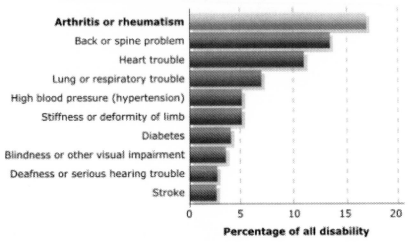

SOURCE: CDC. Prevalence of disability and associated health conditions—United States, 1991–1992. MMWR 1994;43(40): 730–731, 737–739.

The above chart is a sad testament to the true impact it has on our country. Nobody wants to be disabled, yet arthritis is doing that every day. *In fact, one million new patients develop arthritis each year.*[36] With that kind of growth rate, it looks like this chart will grow to an even larger percentage. But other than disabilities, arthritis has many other repercussions. Arthritis results in 39 million physician visits and almost 2.5 million hospitalizations each year.[37] That will surely keep the doctors and hospitals busy and paid in full. On the other hand, it will surely keep the patients busy reaching into and emptying their pocketbooks. But it's not just the patients and their money that is affected. "Arthritis and other rheumatic conditions have an annual economic impact on the nation roughly equivalent to a moderate recession, with an aggregate cost of 1.1 percent of the gross national product", says Edward Yelin, Ph.D., a researcher at the University of California, San Francisco.[38] So, even though the United States is a great country to live in, it doesn't mean that health is automatic.

It is something that needs to be continuously worked at, and perhaps then the health of our country will improve.

14

Summary:
Together We Can Defeat It

It's been over ten years since the start of my health journey. In that time period, I've worked in the mortgage business, the stock market, and even dealt with finance and insurance for the auto industry. Hopefully, in that time span I've helped lower someone's home interest rate, made them some money in the stock market, or even possibly helped them sell some cars. But what has this truly accomplished? It might have helped them financially so they can live a better lifestyle. And yes, having money is important. But is that what's really important in life? Is that what's most important to you? We all know the old saying, "Money can't buy happiness." So let me take this expression to an even higher level by saying that *"Money can't buy long-term health!"* That is what's truly important in life. If you don't have your health, then you don't have much at all. In fact, you could have millions of dollars in the bank, but if you can't get out of bed in the morning due to your illness, then most likely you won't enjoy life, and all your money would be insignificant. That's when it hit me. One day I woke up and realized that I can't let what happened to me go to waste. I had perfect success using these programs, and I couldn't let them go unknown. I am a firm believer that everything happens for a reason in life, and that's why I am writing this book. My ultimate goal is to lead by example, and hopefully the programs I revealed in this book can help you with your current health condition.

There are over 70 million arthritis suffers out there, and I whole-heartedly believe that this book can help each and every one of them. If you are sixty-five years old and reading this book, and you decide that you are only going to try a few of the ideas in this book, that's fantastic. I'm sure the ones you try will help immensely. But if you are a twenty-year old kid and have been diagnosed with an incurable arthritis, the more severe form, then you are facing the same situation that I was in; which was to take drugs and cope with it the rest of your life. This program is ideal for you. *In fact, it is of the utmost importance that you take that leap of faith into the natural world and believe in your body's own healing abilities.* I can assure you that if you are disciplined and follow these programs, you will see great results just as I did. That's my entire reason for writing this book, so that people out there know they have options, and that there is hope for incurable arthritis sufferers. I, too, was in your painful shoes. I was afraid, scared, and confused as to why this was happening in my life. The point I am trying to get across is that if you use common sense and give your body the right healing environment, your body will amaze you and heal just about everything. Remember, your body's number one priority is to survive. Personally, if this book can help just one person defeat their arthritis and rid their body of pain and suffering, then I feel that this book has been a huge success.

You might be thinking to yourselves at this point that this program is too difficult, and that it's all work and no play. You also might be thinking, "I want to have fun in life". Well, it's not fun not being able to walk, or being in excruciating pain every day of your life. Sure, the beginning of this program is not easy, and there are many changes that you must make in your diet and your lifestyle. You have to get used to the idea that your body is in a diseased condition, and that you have to give it special attention. In fact, you have to get used to doing different programs on a daily basis. Once you become accustomed to these changes and start seeing results with the programs, then you will become a solid believer in this program too. You will feel so much healthier and so much more alive that these programs will become second nature to you, and you will never desire to go back to your old eating habits. *It's hard work, but the payout is much greater than the initial sacrifice.* Also, you might be thinking that once you start this program, you will never be able to eat your favorite foods again. You might have the notion that you will be stuck eating veggie burgers, tofu, and salads...and that's it. This is entirely not true! For example, my lifestyle today is much different than it was ten years ago when I was intensely involved in the program. I am definitely not as strict with my food selections as I was way back then. Today, every once in a while I cheat and eat foods that I know are not good for me. I might have some pizza, fried chicken, a frappuccino from Starbuck's, or a piece of candy. But keep in mind that I don't cheat very often. What is even more important are the things that I still do and don't do on a daily basis: I don't take any kind of medications, I don't eat red meat, I don't eat pork products, I don't eat white flour products, I don't eat margarine, I avoid my ten worst foods list as much as possible, etc. Plus, I'm still doing all of the programs in this book because I know that's what my body wants and needs to survive and stay *disease free.* Just remember this before you make your final decision on this program. *Arthritis is not a death-causing disease, but to have a lifetime sentence of pain might be much worse than death itself!*

Okay, so you've now read my book and may be asking yourself, "Why should I believe you; you're not even a doctor?" That's a good question. I know it will be a very hard decision for you to get away from traditional medicine and drugs. Our society has been taught for many years that taking drugs is the only way to go. I'm not asking you to believe in quackery or unproven programs. Everything I have written about in this book is based on facts. I have done all the legwork for you. I have read countless books, journals, articles, and pamphlets. You name it, and I've probably read it. I have gathered research from over 100 different types of professionals, including M.D.'s, Ph.D.'s, Ph.N.'s, N.D.'s, D.C.'s, D.O.'s, R.N.'s, D.D.S.'s, and M.H.A's. I have even used research from Nobel Prize winners. This research comes from highly prestigious medical institutions such as

UCLA, Harvard, Yale, U.C. Berkeley, B.Y.U., Cornell, Tufts, Arizona State, and Loma Linda...so obviously, it can be trusted. It's not just me you are getting this information from; it comes from hundreds of health professionals. I am just passing the information along so that you can use it for your own benefit. Please, look at my bibliography page and read these books. In fact, read as many books as you can, because "knowledge is king". But one thing to be careful of when reading these books is to find out who the author is - or who their sponsor is. If the book is written or sponsored by a pharmaceutical company or a hospital, then obviously it will be biased towards drugs and medicine, not natural products. Once again, from the bottom of my heart, I am asking you to believe the facts. So, if you are thinking about taking the natural approach, and if your current doctor tries to scare you by saying "it's not proven" or "show me the research," put this book in front of him and tell him that I defeated it, and that all the facts he needs are right here. It's important to remember that it's your body, not the doctor's. The last thought I want to leave you with is this: if you can make the wise decision to use the natural programs I've shown in this book, *together we can defeat it!*

Endnotes

Chapter 4   Dr. Marcus Ettinger – The Gerson Program Started

1. Gerson, Max, M.D., *A Cancer Therapy-Results of Fifty Cases*, New York: Station Hill Press, 1997, p 14.

2. Gerson, p. 139.

3. Martin, Raquel, and Romano, Karen J., R.N., D.C, *Preventing and Reversing Arthritis Naturally*, Rochester, Vermont: Healing Arts Press, 2000, p. 16.

4. Kennedy, Ron, M.D., *Nutritional Therapies for Cancer*, 2002, Available at http://www.medical-library.net/sites/_nutritional_therapies_for_cancer.html. Accessed May 28, 2002.

5. Theodosakis, Jason, M.D., M.S., M.P.H., Brenda Adderly, M.H.A., and Barry Fox, Ph.D., *The Arthritis Cure*, New York: St. Martin's Griffin, 1998, p. 114.

6. Sinatra, Stephen T., *Optimum Health*, New York: The Lincoln-Bradley Publishing Group, 1996, p. 209.

7. Gerson, p. 9.

8. Gerson, p. 187.

9. Moss, Ralph, Ph.D., *Detoxification Procedures Archives*, 1998, Available at

http://askwaltstollmd.com/archives/detox.html. Accessed May 31, 2002.

10. Theodosakis, Jason, M.D., M.S., M.P.H., Brenda Adderly, M.H.A., and Barry Fox, Ph.D., *The Arthritis Cure*, New York: St. Martin's Griffin, 1997, p. 112.

11. Matsen, John, N.D., *Mysterious Causes and Cures of Illness,* Ohio: Fischer Publishing Corporation, 1995, p. 28.

12. Matsen, p. 29.

13. Theodosakis et al., *The Arthritis Cure,* p. 3.

14. Gerson, p. 193.

15. Spence, Ted H., DDS, N.D., Ph.D./DSc/M.P.H., *Detoxification, Optimal Wellness Center*, 1997-2002, Available at http://www.mercola.com/1999/oct/10/detoxification.htm Accessed May 28, 2002.

16. Jarvis, D.C., M.D, *Arthritis and Folk Medicine*, New York: Fawcett Crest, 1960, p. 108.

17. Haas, Elson, M.D., *Alternative Medicine, The Definitive Guide*, Washington: Future Medicine Publishing, 1993, p. 157.

18. Welsh, Philip J., D.D.S., N.D., and Leonardo, Bianca, N.D., *Freedom from Arthritis Through Nutrition*, Joshua Tree, California: Tree of Life Publication, 1992, p. 18.

19. Welsh et al., p. 175.

20. Amen, Anusha, R.A., "Sauna Detoxification," *Sacred Space Healing Center*, 2001, Available at http://www.sacredspace-sf.com/saunadetoxification.htm. Accessed May 31, 2002.

21. Null, Gary, Ph.D., Seaman, Barbara, "Detoxification Therapies," *Inner Self Magazine*, 2000, Available at http://www.innerself.com/Magazine/Health/detox003.htm. Accessed May 31, 2002.

22. Moss, Ralph, Ph.D., *Detoxification Procedures Archives*, 1998, Available at http://askwaltstollmd.com/archives/detox.html. Accessed May 31, 2002.

23. Collins, Drew, N.D., *Alternative Medicine, The Definitive Guide*, Washington: Future Medicine Publishing, 1993, p. 143.

24. Collins, Drew, N.D., *Alternative Medicine, The Definitive Guide*, Washington: Future Medicine Publishing, 1993, p. 144.

25. McConnell, Bryan T., N.D., *What are Detoxification/Healing Programs? The First Resort*, Available at http://www.thefirstresortaz.com/home.html. Accessed February 08, 2002.

26. Spence, Ted H., DDS, N.D., Ph.D./DSc/M.P.H., *Detoxification, Optimal Wellness Center*, 1997-2002, Available at http://www.mercola.com/1999/oct/10/detoxification.htm Accessed May 28, 2002.

27. Null, Gary, Ph.D., Seaman, Barbara, "Detoxification Therapies," *Inner Self Magazine*, 2000, Available at

http://www.innerself.com/Magazine/Health/detox003.ht m. Accessed May 31, 2002.

28. Gerson, p. 190.

29. Moss, Ralph, Ph.D., *Detoxification Procedures Archives*, 1998, Available at http://askwaltstollmd.com/archives/detox.html. Accessed May 31, 2002.

30. Ashby, Cheryl, C.C.T., "What are the Benefits of Colon Hydrotherapy?," *The Colon Health Network*, 1997-2002, Available at http://colonhealth.net. Accessed June 04, 2002.

31. Martin, Raquel, and Romano, Karen J., R.N., D.C, *Preventing and Reversing Arthritis Naturally*, Rochester, Vermont: Healing Arts Press, 2000, p. 79.

32. Null, Gary, Ph.D., *Gary Null's Ultimate Lifetime Diet*, New York: Broadway Books, 2000, p. 268.

33. Haas, Elson, M.D., *Alternative Medicine, The Definitive Guide*, Washington: Future Medicine Publishing, 1993, p. 317.

34. Diamond, Harvey and Diamond, Marilyn, *Fit for Life,* New York: Warner Books, 1985, p. 20.

35. Spence, Ted H., DDS, N.D., Ph.D./DSc/M.P.H., *Detoxification, Optimal Wellness Center*, 1997-2002, Available at http://www.mercola.com/1999/oct/10/detoxification.ht m Accessed May 28, 2002.

36. McConnell, Bryan T., N.D., *The First Resort*, Available at http://www.thefirstresortaz.com/home.html. Accessed March 27, 2002.

37.   Gard, Zane, M.D., Brown, Erma, B.S.N., PH. N., *Alternative Medicine, The Definitive Guide*, Washington: Future Medicine Publishing, 1993, p. 303.

38.   Curry, Joel, *Pathways to Health- Why Steam or Sauna*, Available at http://www.pathways2health.net/bensteam.html. Accessed March 27, 2002.

39.   Airola, Paavo, Ph. D., *How to Get Well*, Oregon: Health Press, 1974.

40.   St. Luke's Hospital, *Saunas Linked to Improved Heart Health*, Available at http://yourhealth.stlukesonline.org. Accessed June 6, 2002.

41.   Appleton, Jeremy, N.D., "Saunas Improve Circulation, Reduce Heart Disease Risk," *Healthnotes Newswire*, 2001, Available at http://www.healthnotes.com/online/Back_issues/newswire_2001_10_04_3.htm. Accessed June 27, 2002.

Chapter 5   Dr. Lis Baird – Kinesiology and Herbology Explored

1.   Zampieron, Eugene R., N.D., A.H.G., and Kamhi, Ellen, R.N., H.N.C., *Arthritis: An Alternative Medicine Definitive Guide*, Tiburon, California: AlternativeMedicine.com, 1999, p. 206.

2.   Burton Goldberg Group, *Alternative Medicine, The Definitive Guide*, Washington: Future Medicine Publishing, 1993, p. 47.

3.   Burton Goldberg Group, p. 47.

4.   Burton Goldberg Group, p. 253.

5.   Bove, Mary, N.D., L.M., *Alternative Medicine, The Definitive Guide*, Washington: Future Medicine Publishing, 1993, p. 256.

6.   Weil, Andrew, M.D., *Alternative Medicine, The Definitive Guide*, Washington: Future Medicine Publishing, 1993, p. 255.

7.   Balch, James F., M.D., and Phyllis A. Balch, C.N.C, *Prescription for Nutritional Healing*, Garden City Park, New York: Avery Publishing Group, 1997, p. 49.

8.   Mindell, Earl, R.Ph., Ph.D., *Earl Mindell's Food as Medicine*, New York: Simon & Schuster, 1994, p. 87.

9.   *Cayenne*, Available at http://www.gardenguides.com/herbs/cayenne.htm. Accessed June 29, 2002.

10.   *Cayenne*, Available at http://www.gardenguides.com/herbs/cayenne.htm. Accessed June 29, 2002.

11.   *Cayenne*, Available at http://www.gardenguides.com/herbs/cayenne.htm. Accessed June 29, 2002.

12.   Mindell, p. 115.

13.   "Devil's Claw for Osteoarthritis," *Positive Health Complementary Medicine Magazine*, 1994-2002, Available at http://www.positivehealth.com/Reviews/osteo58.htm. Accessed June 29, 2002.

14. Brown, Donald J., *Herbal Prescriptions for Better Health*, Rocklin, California: Prima Publishing, 1995, p. 267.

15. "Devil's Claw for Osteoarthritis," *Positive Health Complementary Medicine Magazine*, 1994-2002, Available at http://www.positivehealth.com/Reviews/osteo58.htm. Accessed June 29, 2002.

16. Chantre P., Cappelaere A., Leblan D., "Efficacy and tolerance of Harpagophytum procumbens versus diacerhein in treatment of osteoarthritis," Phytomedicine 2000, 7(3): 177-183.

17. Horner, Christine, M.D., *Natural Headache Relief: Feverfew*, Available at http://www.channelcincinnati.com/cin/health/healthtea m/stories.htm. Accessed June 29, 2002.

18. Foster, Steven, *Feverfew*, 2000, Available at http://www.stevenfoster.com/education/monograph/feve rfew.html. Accessed June 29, 2002.

19. Horner, Christine, M.D., *Natural Headache Relief: Feverfew*, Available at http://www.channelcincinnati.com/cin/health/healthtea m/stories.htm. Accessed June 29, 2002.

20. Carper, Jean, *Food Your Miracle Medicine*, New York: Harper Collins Publishers, 1993, p. 340.

21. Borek, Carmia, Ph.D., *Garlic-The Bountiful Bulb,* 1995-2002, Available at http://www.lef.org/magazine/mag2000/jan00-report1.html. Accessed April 04, 2002.

22. Borek, Carmia, Ph.D., *Garlic-The Bountiful Bulb,* 1995-2002, Available at

http://www.lef.org/magazine/mag2000/jan00-report1.html. Accessed April 04, 2002.

23. Carper, p. 340.

24. Spence, Ted H., DDS, N.D., Ph.D./DSc/M.P.H., *Detoxification, Optimal Wellness Center*, 1997-2002, Available at http://www.mercola.com/1999/oct/10/detoxification.ht m Accessed May 28, 2002.

25. Lau, Benjamin, M.D., *Garlic for Health*, Wilmot, Wisconsin: Lotus Light Publications, 1988, p. 25.

26. Carper, p. 73.

27. Carattini, Lisa, *Nutritional Benefits of Ginger*, Available at http://okok.essortment.com/benefitsginger_rahr.htm. Accessed June 24, 2002.

28. Carattini, Lisa, *Nutritional Benefits of Ginger*, Available at http://okok.essortment.com/benefitsginger_rahr.htm. Accessed June 24, 2002.

29. Carper, p. 382.

30. Srivastava, K.C., Mustafa, T., "Ginger in rheumatism and musculoskeletal disorders," *Department of Environmental Medicine*, Odense University, Denmark, Med. Hypotheses 39, 1992, pp. 342-348.

31. Decker, Elizabeth, "Detox Your Liver with Milk Thistle," *Robeks,* 2002, Available at http://www.robeks.com. Accessed July 5, 2002.

32. Decker, Elizabeth, "Detox Your Liver with Milk Thistle," *Robeks,* 2002, Available at http://www.robeks.com. Accessed July 5, 2002.

33. Castleman, Michael, "Milk Thistle: Nature's Liver Protector," *Earthpharmacy*, 2001, Available at http://www.earthpharmacy.com/milkthistlearticle.html. Accessed July 5, 2002.

34. Castleman, Michael, "Milk Thistle: Nature's Liver Protector," *Earthpharmacy*, 2001, Available at http://www.earthpharmacy.com/milkthistlearticle.html. Accessed July 5, 2002.

35. "Milk Thistle: Protection for the Liver," *Herba-Medica*, 2001, Available at http://www.herba-medica.com/remedies/milkthistle.html. Accessed July 5, 2002.

36. Barclay, Laurie, "Liver Detoxification-Fact or Fad?" *WebMD*, 1996-2002, Available at http://webmd.lycos.com/content/article/1685.52520. Accessed July 5, 2002.

37. Bisset, N.G., "Salicis Cortex: Willow Bark," in *Herbal Drugs and Pyhtopharmaceuticals: A Handbook for Practice on a Scientific Basis*, Stuttgart: Medpharm Scientific Publishers, 1994, pp. 437-439.

38. "White Willow Bark", *WholeHealthMD.com*, Available at http://www.wholehealthmd.com/refshelf/substances_view/1,1525,10069,00.html. Accessed May 20, 2002.

39. Law, Ron, *Safety of Dietary Supplements*, Available at http://www.laleva.cc/petizione/english/ronlaw_eng.html. Accessed June 28,2002.

40. Airola, Paavo O., N.D., *There is a Cure for Arthritis*, West Nyack, New York: Parker Publishing Company, 1968, p. 35.

41. "White Willow", *OrganicFood.co.uk*, Available at http:// www.organicfood.co.uk/herbs/whitewillow.html. Accessed June 5, 2002.

42. *YUCCALIVE*, Available at http://www.mpsmarketing.com/YuccaliveInfo.htm. Accessed June 29, 2002.

43. *YUCCALIVE*, Available at http://www.mpsmarketing.com/YuccaliveInfo.htm. Accessed June 29, 2002.

Chapter 6 Gary Richer – The Live Cell King

1. Christianson, Kent, Dr., "Live Blood Cell Analysis," *Holistic Chiropractic and Healing Arts Center*, Available at: http://www.drkent.com/analysis.html. Accessed June 6, 2002.

2. Mercola, Joseph, D.O., "Live Cell Analysis," *Optimal Wellness Center*, 1997-2002, Available at http://www.mercola.com. Accessed June 6, 2002.

3. Rona, Zoltan, M.D., *Live Cell Microscopy- Window to a Hidden World,* 1999-2002, Available at: http://www.healthwatcher.net. Accessed June 6, 2002.

4. *Cayenne -The Super Herb*, Available at http://www.formulamaster.com/cayenne.htm. Accessed June 29, 2002.

5. Jarvis, D.C., M.D, *Arthritis and Folk Medicine*, New York: Fawcett Crest, 1960, p. 103.

6. Jarvis, D.C., M.D, *Arthritis and Folk Medicine*, New York: Fawcett Crest, 1960, p. 126.

7.   Diamond, Harvey and Diamond, Marilyn, *Fit for Life,* New York: Warner Books, 1985, p. 41.

8.   Lee, Thomas F., Ph.D., *Conquering Rheumatoid Arthritis*, New York: Prometheus Books, 2001, p. 122.

9.   Jarvis, p. 126.

10. Matsen, John, N.D., *Mysterious Causes and Cures of Illness,* Ohio: Fischer Publishing Corporation, 1995, p. 94.

11. Matsen, John, N.D., *Mysterious Causes and Cures of Illness,* Ohio: Fischer Publishing Corporation, 1995, p. 58.

12. Matsen, John, N.D., *Mysterious Causes and Cures of Illness,* Ohio: Fischer Publishing Corporation, 1995, p. 160.

13. Mercola, Joseph, D.O., "Live Cell Analysis," *Optimal Wellness Center*, 1997-2002, Available at http://www.mercola.com. Accessed June 6, 2002.

14. Horne, Steven H., *Constitutional Iridology*, Utah: Tree of Light Institute, Inc., 1997, p. 2-4.

15. Matsen, pp. 83-84.

Chapter 7   Dr. Terry Pfau – Homeopathic Help from Las Vegas

1.   Burton Goldberg Group, *Alternative Medicine, The Definitive Guide*, Washington: Future Medicine Publishing, 1993, p. 272.

2.   Ivker, Robert S., D.O., and Nelson, Todd, N.D., *Arthritis Survival, The Holistic Medical Treatment Program for Osteoarthritis*, New York: Penguin Putnam, Inc., 2001, p. 68.

3.   Matsen, John, N.D., *Mysterious Causes and Cures of Illness,* Ohio: Fischer Publishing Corporation, 1995, p. 284.

4.   Ullman, Dana, M.P.H, *A Modern Understanding of Homeopathic Medicine*, 1991, Available at http://www.homeopathic.com/intro/modern.htm. Accessed February 08, 2002.

5.   Anderson-Parrado, Patricia, "Homeopathic Remedies to Ease Acute and Chronic Arthritis Pain," *Better Nutrition* 159, no. 2, February 1997: 26.

6.   Ulman, Dana, M.P.H., *Homeopathy Medicine for the 21st Century*, Berkeley, California: North Atlantic Books, 1988, p. 165.

7.   Burton Goldberg Group, *Alternative Medicine, The Definitive Guide*, Washington: Future Medicine Publishing, 1993, p. 276.

Chapter 8   Other Natural Supplements – Immune System Boosters

1.   Mindell, Earl, R.Ph., Ph.D., *Earl Mindell's Food as Medicine*, New York: Simon & Schuster, 1994, p. 9.

2.   Barefoot, Robert R., *Death by Diet*, Southeastern, Pennsylvania: Triad Marketing, 2002, p. 25.

3.   DeCava, Judith A., *The Real Truth about Vitamins and Antioxidants*, Columbus, Georgia: Brentwood Academic Press, 1996, p. 160.

4.   Balch, James F., M.D., and Phyllis A. Balch, C.N.C, *Prescription for Nutritional Healing*, Garden City Park, New York: Avery Publishing Group, 1997, pp. 12-13.

5.   *Multi-Vitamin/Mineral*, Available at http://www.sbwise.com/healthinfo/Multivitamin.htm. Accessed June 29, 2002.

6.   Belanger, James T., N.D., "How to Select a Good Multivitamin for Your Family," *Lexington Natural Health Center*, Available at http://home1.gte.net/res03kui/pages/VitaminsArt.html. Accessed June 27, 2002.

7.   Balch et al., p. 13.

8.   Balch et al., p. 13.

9.   *Multi-Vitamin/Mineral*, Available at http://www.sbwise.com/healthinfo/Multivitamin.htm. Accessed June 29, 2002.

10.   "DDS Acidophilus," *HSR Magazine*, 2002, Available at http://www.hsrmagazine.com/articles/191brand1.html. Accessed July 5, 2002.

11.   Challem, Jack, "Is Alpha-Lipoic Acid the 'Ideal' Antioxidant?" *ImmuneAlive Education*, Available at http://www.immunalive.com/alpha-lipoic_acid.html. Accessed June 29, 2002.

12. "Alpha-Lipoic Acid," *Wellness Guide to Dietary Supplements*, 2002, Available at http://www.berkeleywellness.com. Accessed June 29, 2002.

13. Schmid, Ron, N.D., *Alpha lipoic Acid - the Universal Antioxidant That Saves Lives*, 2002, Available at http://www.DrRons.com. Accessed June 29, 2002.

14. *Alpha Lipoic Acid and HCV*, 2000, Available at http://www.objectivemedicine.com/sample2antioxidant.htm. Accessed June 29. 2002.

15. Sahelian, Ray, M.D., and Byrd, Edward, *Lipoic Acid: The Unique Antioxidant*, Available at http://www.bodybuilding.com/store/ala.html. Accessed June 29, 2002.

16. Jarvis, D.C., M.D, *Arthritis and Folk Medicine*, New York: Fawcett Crest, 1960, p. 130.

17. Jarvis, D.C., M.D, *Arthritis and Folk Medicine*, New York: Fawcett Crest, 1960, p. 127.

18. Bragg, Paul C., and Bragg, Patricia, *Apple Cider Vinegar Health System*, Santa Barbara, California: Health Science, 1992, pp. 26-29.

19. "Bromelain," *Health Journal*, Available at http://www.bodyandfitness.com/Information/Health/Research/bromelain.htm. Accessed June 25, 2002.

20. Theodosakis, Jason, M.D., M.S., M.P.H., Brenda Adderly, M.H.A., and Barry Fox, Ph.D., *Maximizing the Arthritis Cure*, New York: St. Martin's Griffin, 1998, p. 211.

21. Meinig, George E., DDS, FACD, "Bromelain," *Price-Pottenger Nutrition Foundation,* 1997-1999, Available at http://www.price-pottenger.org/Articles/Bromelain.html. Accessed June 25, 2002.

22. "Bromelain," *Health Journal,* Available at http://www.bodyandfitness.com/Information/Health/Research/bromelain.htm. Accessed June 25, 2002.

23. "The Omega Zone," *ABC News,* 2002, Available at http://abcnews.go.com/sections/community/DailyNews/chat_omegazone050802.html. Accessed July 5, 2002.

24. "Cod Liver Oil Benefits Confirmed," *BBC News,* Available at http://news.bbc.co.uk/hi/english/health/newsid_1817000/1817974.stm. Accessed July 5, 2002.

25. Mindell, pp. 27-28.

26. Williams, David, "Dangers of Alternative Medicine, " *The Worldwide Journal of Lifelong Health,* Fall 1998, p. 95.

27. Balch et al., p. 51.

28. Edelson, Stephen B., M.D., F.A.A.F.P., F.A.A.E.M., *Scientific Studies of MSM,* 2002, Available at http://www.oralchelation.com/methyl/data/data7.htm. Accessed May 29, 2002.

29. Muir, Maya, *DMSO: Many Uses, Much Controversy,* 2001-2002, Available at http://www.dmso.org/articles/information/muir.htm. Accessed April 09, 2002.

30. Whitaker, Julian, "DMSO Protects the Spine in Acute Phase," *Dr. Julian Whitaker's Health and Healing* (supplement), May 1998, pp. 1-2.

31. "Why Enzymes?" *Lifestar*, Available at http://www.lifestar.com/Pages/WhyEnzymes1.html. Accessed June 26, 2002.

32. "Why Enzymes?" *Lifestar*, Available at http://www.lifestar.com/Pages/WhyEnzymes1.html. Accessed June 26, 2002.

33. Balch et al., p. 47.

34. Heath, Allison, "Food Enzymes - A Key to Unlocking Our Health", *Celltech*, 2002, Available at http://www.celltech.com/resources/technical/Enzymes_Aheath.asp. Accessed July 5, 2002.

35. Ali, Majid, M.D., *The Ghoraa and Limbic Exercise*, Denville, New Jersey: IPM Press, 1993, p. 94.

36. Lipski, Elizabeth, M.S., C.C.N., *Digestive Wellness, Second Edition*, 2000, pp. 220-221.

37. Heath, Allison, "Food Enzymes - A Key to Unlocking Our Health", *Celltech*, 2002, Available at http://www.celltech.com/resources/technical/Enzymes_Aheath.asp. Accessed July 5, 2002.

38. Murray, Michael T., "Irrefutable Evidence: Glucosamine Sulfate Proven Superior Over Other Forms of Glucosamine and Chondroitin Sulfate," *Vitale Communication* (brochure), 30 May 1997.

39. Theodosakis et al., p. 21.

40. Theodosakis et al., p. 22.

41.   Martin, Raquel, and Romano, Karen J., R.N., D.C, *Preventing and Reversing Arthritis Naturally*, Rochester, Vermont: Healing Arts Press, 2000, p. 19.

42.   Fox, Barry, Ph.D., *Arthritis for Dummies*, New York: Hungry Minds, Inc., 2000, p. 152.

43.   "JAMA Meta-analysis finds Glucosamine and Chondroitin Useful for Arthritis," *Associated Press*, March 15, 2000, Available at http://www.herbs.org/current/JAMA-glucosamine.html. Accessed June 29, 2002.

44.   Walker, Morton, D.P.M., "The Nutritional Therapeutics of Masquelier's Oligomeric ProanthoCyanidins (OPCs), "*LifePlusVitamins*, Available at http://www.lifeplusvitamins.com/articlewalker.htm. Accessed July 5, 2002.

45.   Hansen, Clark, N.D., "Grape Seed Extract: GSE 50 & GSE 100," *Nutracor*, Available at http://www.nutracor.com/hcc/hcc_gse.html. Accessed July 5, 2002.

46.   Hansen, Clark, N.D., "Grape Seed Extract: GSE 50 & GSE 100," *Nutracor*, Available at http://www.nutracor.com/hcc/hcc_gse.html. Accessed July 5, 2002.

47.   Schmid, Ron, N.D., "Grape Seed Extract - A Powerful Antioxidant with Wide Ranging Benefits," *Dr. Rons*, 2002, Available at http://www.drrons.com/grape_seed_extract.html. Accessed July 5, 2002.

48.   Oldenburg, Ann, *USA Today - Coburn beats back tough disease*, Available at

http://www.bulkmsm.com/research/JamesCoburn/james6.htm. Accessed May 29, 2002.

49. Oldenburg, Ann, *USA Today - Coburn beats back tough disease*, Available at http://www.bulkmsm.com/research/JamesCoburn/james6.htm. Accessed May 29, 2002.

50. Oldenburg, Ann, *USA Today - Coburn beats back tough disease*, Available at http://www.bulkmsm.com/research/JamesCoburn/james6.htm. Accessed May 29, 2002.

51. Jacob, Stanley W., M.D., *MSM, What the Doctors Say about MSM*, Available at http://www.a1msm.co.uk/009_doctors/01_what_the_doctors_say_about_msm.htm. Accessed May 29, 2002.

52. *MSM Overview, Integrative Research*, 2001, Available at http://www.integrativeresearch.com/72137/msm/Overview/msmoverview.htm. Accessed May 29, 2002.

53. Jacob, Stanley W., M.D., *MSM, What the Doctors Say about MSM*, Available at http://www.a1msm.co.uk/009_doctors/01_what_the_doctors_say_about_msm.htm. Accessed May 29, 2002.

54. Lawrence, Ronald, M.D., Ph.D., "Methylsulfonyl-methane (M.S.M.): A Double-Blind Study of Its Use in Degenerative Arthritis," *International Journal of Anti-Aging Medicine* 1, no.1 (1998): 50.

55. "What are the Benefits of Potassium," *Lifeclinic*, Available at http://lifeclinic.com. Accessed July 5, 2002.

56. Wade, Carlson, *Inner Cleansing - How to Free Yourself From Joint-Muscle-Artery-Circulation Sludge*, West

Nyack, New York: Parker Publishing Company, 1992, p. 51.

57. Carper, Jean, *Food Your Miracle Medicine*, New York: Harper Collins Publishers, 1993, p. 100.

58. Carper, Jean, *Food Your Miracle Medicine*, New York: Harper Collins Publishers, 1993, p. 89.

59. Pauling, Linus, *How to Live Longer and Feel Better*, New York: W.H. Freeman and Company, 1986, p. 8.

60. Cameron, Ewan, and Pauling, Linus, *Cancer and Vitamin C*, Menlo Park, California: Linus Pauling Institute of Science and Medicine, 1979, p. 100.

61. Cameron, Ewan, and Pauling, Linus, *Cancer and Vitamin C*, Menlo Park, California: Linus Pauling Institute of Science and Medicine, 1979, p. 101.

62. Mindell, p. 55.

63. Null, Gary, Ph.D., *Gary Null's Ultimate Lifetime Diet*, New York: Broadway Books, 2000, p. 288.

64. Mindell, p. 56.

65. Spence, Ted H., DDS, N.D., Ph.D./DSc/M.P.H., *Detoxification, Optimal Wellness Center*, 1997-2002, Available at http://www.mercola.com/1999/oct/10/detoxification.htm Accessed May 28, 2002.

66. Fox, Barry, Ph.D., *Arthritis for Dummies*, New York: Hungry Minds, Inc., 2000, p. 148.

67. Wade, Carlson, *Inner Cleansing- How to Free Yourself From Joint-Muscle-Artery-Circulation Sludge*, West

Nyack, New York: Parker Publishing Company, 1992, pp. 139-140.

68. "Do You Need More 'E'?" *Tufts E-news*, 2001, Available at http://enews.tufts.edu/stories/053102NeedMoreE.htm. Accessed July 2, 2002.

69. *Scientists are won Over by the Benefits of Supplements*, 1999-2002, Available at http://www.nutritionfocus.com. Accessed June 29, 2002.

70. Howard, Sharon, R.D., "Benefits of Vitamin E," *drkoop*, 1998-2001, Available at http://www.drkoop.com/wellness/nutrition/vitiamins_mi nerals/index226.html. Accessed July 2, 2002.

71. *Scientists are won Over by the Benefits of Supplements*, 1999-2002, Available at http://www.nutritionfocus.com. Accessed June 29, 2002.

72. Passwater, Richard A, Ph.D., "Vitamin E's Health Benefits Beyond Those of Correcting Deficiency," *Nutrition Focus*, 2001, Available at http://www.nutritionfocus.com/nutrition_library/machli n_interview.html. Accessed July 2, 2002.

73. Salvatore, Steve, M.D., "Vitamin E may Reduce Risk of Stroke," *CNN Interactive*, 2001, Available at http://www.cnn.com/HEALTH/9904/20/vitamin.e.strok e/. Accessed July 2, 2002.

74. *Scientists are won Over by the Benefits of Supplements*, 1999-2002, Available at http://www.nutritionfocus.com. Accessed June 29, 2002.

75. Mindell, p. 61.

76. *Scientists are won Over by the Benefits of Supplements*, 1999-2002, Available at http://www.nutritionfocus.com. Accessed June 29, 2002.

Chapter 10 Arthritis Stopped – My Immune System Wins

1. Jarvis, D.C., M.D, *Arthritis and Folk Medicine*, New York: Fawcett Crest, 1960, p. 128.

2. Cousins, Norman, *Anatomy of an Illness As Perceived by the Patient*, New York: W.W. Norton & Company, 1979, p. 11.

3. Airola, Paavo O., N.D., *There is a Cure for Arthritis*, West Nyack, New York: Parker Publishing Company, 1968, p. 53.

4. Martin, Raquel, and Romano, Karen J., R.N., D.C, *Preventing and Reversing Arthritis Naturally*, Rochester, Vermont: Healing Arts Press, 2000, p. 11.

5. Jarvis, D.C., M.D., p. 76.

6. Airola, Paavo O., N.D., p. 42.

7. Ullman, Dana, M.P.H, *A Modern Understanding of Homeopathic Medicine*, 1991, Available at http://www.homeopathic.com/intro/modern.htm. Accessed February 08, 2002.

8. Matsen, John, N.D., *Mysterious Causes and Cures of Illness,* Ohio: Fischer Publishing Corporation, 1995, p. 95.

9.   Diamond, Harvey and Diamond, Marilyn, *Fit for Life II: Living Health -The Complete Health Program,* New York: Warner Books, 1987, p. 63.

10.   Diamond, Harvey and Diamond, Marilyn, *Fit for Life II: Living Health -The Complete Health Program,* New York: Warner Books, 1987, p. 63.

11.   Laux, Marcus, N.D., *Is "Modern" Medicine Killing You?* Potomac, Maryland: Dr. Marcus Laux's Naturally Well, 1995, p. 28.

12.   Appleton, Jeremy, N.D., "Breathe Easier: Antioxidants Protect Lungs from Ozone Damage," *Healthnotes Newswire,* 1998-2002, Available at http://www.healthnotes.com/online/Back_issues/newswire_2001_11_21_1.htm. Accessed June 27, 2002.

13.   Ivker, Robert S., D.O., and Nelson, Todd, N.D., *Arthritis Survival, The Holistic Medical Treatment Program for Osteoarthritis,* New York: Penguin Putnam, Inc., 2001, p. 93.

14.   Martin, Raquel, and Romano, Karen J., R.N., D.C, *Preventing and Reversing Arthritis Naturally,* Rochester, Vermont: Healing Arts Press, 2000, p. 34.

15.   Martin, Raquel, and Romano, Karen J., R.N., D.C, p. 34-35.

16.   Balch, James F., M.D., and Phyllis A. Balch, C.N.C, *Prescription for Nutritional Healing,* Garden City Park, New York: Avery Publishing Group, 1997, p. 30.

17.   Diamond, Harvey and Diamond, Marilyn, *Fit for Life II: Living Health -The Complete Health Program,* New York: Warner Books, 1987, p. 98.

18. Balch, James F., M.D., and Phyllis A. Balch, C.N.C, *Prescription for Nutritional Healing*, Garden City Park, New York: Avery Publishing Group, 1997, p. 30.

19. Diamond, Harvey and Diamond, Marilyn, *Fit for Life II: Living Health -The Complete Health Program,* New York: Warner Books, 1987, p. 103.

20. Balch, James F., M.D., and Phyllis A. Balch, C.N.C, *Prescription for Nutritional Healing*, Garden City Park, New York: Avery Publishing Group, 1997, p. 31.

21. Martin, Raquel, and Romano, Karen J., R.N., D.C, *Preventing and Reversing Arthritis Naturally*, Rochester, Vermont: Healing Arts Press, 2000, p. 35.

22. Diamond, Harvey and Diamond, Marilyn, *Fit for Life II: Living Health -The Complete Health Program,* New York: Warner Books, 1987, p. 101.

23. "Acidophilus," *Nutrition Now, Inc.*, 1995-2002, Available at http://www.nutritionnow.com/acidoinf.htm. Accessed July 5, 2002.

24. Matsen, John, N.D., p. 15.

25. Erasmus, Udo, *Fats that Heal, Fats that Kill*, Vancouver, B.C., Canada: Alive Books, 1997, p. 355.

26. Diamond, Harvey and Diamond, Marilyn, *Fit for Life,* New York: Warner Books, 1985, p. 63.

27. Spence, Ted H., DDS, N.D., Ph.D./DSc/M.P.H., *Detoxification, Optimal Wellness Center*, 1997-2002, Available at http://www.mercola.com/1999/oct/10/detoxification.htm Accessed May 28, 2002.

28. Matsen, John, N.D., p. 163.

29. Donsbach, Kurt W., D.C., N.D., Ph.D., and Alsleben, H. Rudolph, M.D., D.O., Ph.D., *Arthritis Wholistic Therapy*, Al-Don Institute of Experimental Medicine, 1992, p. 64.

30. "The Importance of Food Enzymes," *Celltech*, 2002, Available at http://www.celltech.com/resources/technical/Importanc e_of_enzymes.asp. Accessed July 5, 2002.

31. Matsen, John, N.D., p. 114.

32. Matsen, John, N.D., p. 118.

33. Matsen, John, N.D., p. 25.

34. Martin, Raquel, and Romano, Karen J., R.N., D.C, *Preventing and Reversing Arthritis Naturally*, Rochester, Vermont: Healing Arts Press, 2000, p. 51.

35. Martin, Raquel, and Romano, Karen J., R.N., D.C, p. 51.

36. Chopra, Deepak, M.D., *Ageless Body Timeless Mind*, New York: Harmony Books, 1993, p. 124.

37. Wade, Carlson, *Inner Cleansing - How to Free Yourself From Joint-Muscle-Artery-Circulation Sludge*, West Nyack, New York: Parker Publishing Company, 1992, p. 10.

38. Lane, Nancy E., M.D., and Wallace, Danielle J., M.D., *All About Osteoarthritis, The Definitive Resource for Arthritis Patients and their Families*, New York: Oxford University Press, 2002, p. 182.

39. Murray, Michael T., N.D., *Natural Alternatives to Over-the-Counter and Prescription Drugs*, New York: William Morrow and Company Inc., 1994, p. 275.

40. Null, Gary, Ph.D., Seaman, Barbara, "Detoxification Therapies," *Inner Self Magazine*, 2000, Available at http://www.innerself.com/Magazine/Health/detox003.htm. Accessed May 31, 2002.

41. Matsen, John, N.D., p. 157.

42. Martin, Raquel, and Romano, Karen J., R.N., D.C, *Preventing and Reversing Arthritis Naturally*, Rochester, Vermont: Healing Arts Press, 2000, p. 32.

43. Theodosakis, Jason, M.D., M.S., M.P.H., Brenda Adderly, M.H.A., and Barry Fox, Ph.D., *The Arthritis Cure*, New York: St. Martin's Griffin, 1997, p. 82.

44. Theodosakis, Jason, M.D., M.S., M.P.H., p. 82.

45. Lane, Nancy E., M.D., and Wallace, Danielle J., M.D., *All About Osteoarthritis, The Definitive Resource for Arthritis Patients and their Families*, New York: Oxford University Press, 2002, p. 123.

46. Fox, Barry, Ph.D., *Arthritis for Dummies*, New York: Hungry Minds, Inc., 2000, p. 207.

47. Welsh, Philip J., D.D.S., N.D., and Leonardo, Bianca, N.D., *Freedom from Arthritis Through Nutrition*, Joshua Tree, California: Tree of Life Publication, 1992, p. 193.

48. Laux, Marcus, N.D., *Is "Modern" Medicine Killing You?* Potomac, Maryland: Dr. Marcus Laux's Naturally Well, 1995, p. 89.

Chapter 11 Food Choices – What's Good, What's Bad

1. Kane, Emily, N.D., *Enzymes: The Difference between Raw and Cooked Foods*, Available at http://www.heathly.net/asp/templates/article.asp. Accessed June 26, 2002.

2. Mindell, Earl, R.Ph., Ph.D., *Earl Mindell's Food as Medicine*, New York: Simon & Schuster, 1994, p. 13.

3. Airola, Paavo O., N.D., *There is a Cure for Arthritis*, West Nyack, New York: Parker Publishing Company, 1968, p. 64.

4. Williams, David G., *Alternatives*, Rockville, Maryland: Mountain Home Publishing, 2002, p. 6.

5. Mindell, Earl, R.Ph., Ph.D., *Earl Mindell's Food as Medicine*, New York: Simon & Schuster, 1994, p. 10.

6. Donsbach, Kurt W., *Arthritis*, Rosarito Beach, Baja, California: Wholistic Publications, 1981, p. 3.

7. Null, Gary, Ph.D., *Gary Null's Ultimate Lifetime Diet*, New York: Broadway Books, 2000, p. 144.

8. Airola, Paavo O., N.D., *There is a Cure for Arthritis*, West Nyack, New York: Parker Publishing Company, 1968, p. 43-44.

9. *Multi-Vitamin/Mineral*, Available at http://www.sbwise.com/healthinfo/Multivitamin.htm. Accessed June 29, 2002.

10. Welsh, Philip J., D.D.S., N.D., and Leonardo, Bianca, N.D., *Freedom from Arthritis Through Nutrition*,

Joshua Tree, California: Tree of Life Publication, 1992, p. 46.

11. Diamond, Harvey and Diamond, Marilyn, *Fit for Life II: Living Health -The Complete Health Program,* New York: Warner Books, 1987, p. 324.

12. Mullins, Eustace, *Murder by Injection: The Story of the Medical Conspiracy Against America*, Staunton, Virginia: The National Council for Medical Research, 1988, p. 214.

13. Murray, Michael T., N.D., *Natural Alternatives to Over-the-Counter and Prescription Drugs*, New York: William Morrow and Company Inc., 1994, p. 22.

14. Welsh, Philip J., D.D.S., N.D., and Leonardo, Bianca, N.D., *Freedom from Arthritis Through Nutrition,* Joshua Tree, California: Tree of Life Publication, 1992, p. 215.

15. Laux, Marcus, N.D., *Is "Modern" Medicine Killing You?* Potomac, Maryland: Dr. Marcus Laux's Naturally Well, 1995, p. 32.

16. Fallon, Sally W., and Enig, Mary G., "Why Butter is Better," *Health Freedom News* 14, no. 6, November/December 1995: 12-14.

17. Diamond, Harvey and Diamond, Marilyn, *Fit for Life,* New York: Warner Books, 1985, p. 110.

18. Diamond, Harvey and Diamond, Marilyn, *Fit for Life,* New York: Warner Books, 1985, p. 109.

19. Diamond, Harvey and Diamond, Marilyn, *Fit for Life,* New York: Warner Books, 1985, p. 111.

20. Carper, Jean, *Food Your Miracle Medicine*, New York: Harper Collins Publishers, 1993, p. 353.

21. Carper, Jean, *Food Your Miracle Medicine*, New York: Harper Collins Publishers, 1993, p. 156.

22. Carper, Jean, *Food Your Miracle Medicine*, New York: Harper Collins Publishers, 1993, p. 173.

23. Carper, Jean, *Food Your Miracle Medicine*, New York: Harper Collins Publishers, 1993, p. 224.

24. Carper, Jean, *Food Your Miracle Medicine*, New York: Harper Collins Publishers, 1993, p. 211.

25. Jarvis, D.C., M.D, *Arthritis and Folk Medicine*, New York: Fawcett Crest, 1960, p. 44.

26. Margen, Sheldon, M.D., and the Editors of the University of California at Berkeley Wellness Letter, *The Wellness Encyclopedia of Food and Nutrition*, New York: Random House, 1992, p. 305.

27. Donsbach, Kurt W., D.C., N.D., Ph.D., and Alsleben, H. Rudolph, M.D., D.O., Ph.D., *Arthritis Wholistic Therapy*, Al-Don Institute of Experimental Medicine, 1992, p. 61.

28. Martin, Raquel, and Romano, Karen J., R.N., D.C, *Preventing and Reversing Arthritis Naturally*, Rochester, Vermont: Healing Arts Press, 2000, p. 43.

29. Carper, Jean, *Food Your Miracle Medicine*, New York: Harper Collins Publishers, 1993, p. 13.

30. Carper, Jean, *Food Your Miracle Medicine*, New York: Harper Collins Publishers, 1993, p. 381-382.

31. Carper, Jean, *Food Your Miracle Medicine*, New York: Harper Collins Publishers, 1993, p. 35.

32. Mindell, Earl, R.Ph., Ph.D., *Earl Mindell's Food as Medicine*, New York: Simon & Schuster, 1994, p. 145.

33. Carper, Jean, *Food Your Miracle Medicine*, New York: Harper Collins Publishers, 1993, p. 91.

34. Carper, Jean, *Food Your Miracle Medicine*, New York: Harper Collins Publishers, 1993, p. 35.

35. Wade, Carlson, *Inner Cleansing - How to Free Yourself From Joint-Muscle-Artery-Circulation Sludge*, West Nyack, New York: Parker Publishing Company, 1992, p. 6.

36. Donsbach, Kurt W., D.C., N.D., Ph.D., and Alsleben, H. Rudolph, M.D., D.O., Ph.D., *Arthritis Wholistic Therapy*, Al-Don Institute of Experimental Medicine, 1992, p. 67.

37. Weil, Andrew, M.D., *Natural Health, Natural Medicine*, New York: Houghton Mifflin Company, 1995, p. 322.

38. Airola, Paavo O., *There is a Cure for Arthritis*, West Nyack, New York: Parker Publishing Company, 1968, p. 73.

39. Carper, Jean, *Food Your Miracle Medicine*, New York: Harper Collins Publishers, 1993, p. 37.

40. Carper, Jean, *Food Your Miracle Medicine*, New York: Harper Collins Publishers, 1993, p. 243.

41. Diamond, Harvey and Diamond, Marilyn, *Fit for Life: Living Health -The Complete Health Program,* New York: Warner Books, 1985, p. 125-126.

42. Balch, James F., M.D., and Phyllis A. Balch, C.N.C, *Prescription for Nutritional Healing,* Garden City Park, New York: Avery Publishing Group, 1997, p. 9.

43. Monte, Woodrow C., "Aspartame: Methanol and the Public Health," *Journal of Applied Nutrition* 36, no. 1, November 1984: p. 41-52.

44. Gerson, Max, M.D., p. 14.

45. Gerson, Max, M.D., p. 151.

46. Jarvis, D.C., M.D, *Arthritis and Folk Medicine,* New York: Fawcett Crest, 1960, p. 44.

47. Gerson, Max, M.D., p. 151.

48. Laux, Marcus, N.D., *Is "Modern" Medicine Killing You?* Potomac, Maryland: Dr. Marcus Laux's Naturally Well, 1995, p. 24.

49. Airola, Paavo O., N.D., *There is a Cure for Arthritis,* West Nyack, New York: Parker Publishing Company, 1968, p. 61.

50. Null, Gary, Ph.D., *Gary Null's Ultimate Lifetime Diet,* New York: Broadway Books, 2000, p. 159.

51. Whitaker, Julian, "Stanford No Longer Used Microwaves to Warm Breast Milk," *Dr. Julian Whitaker's Health and Healing* 3, no. 9, September 1993: 3.

52. Spence, Ted H., DDS, N.D., Ph.D./DSc/M.P.H., *Detoxification, Optimal Wellness Center,* 1997-2002, Avail-

able at
http://www.mercola.com/1999/oct/10/detoxification.ht
m Accessed May 28, 2002.

53. Balch, James F., M.D., and Phyllis A. Balch, C.N.C,
     Prescription for Nutritional Healing, Garden City Park,
     New York: Avery Publishing Group, 1997, p. 124.

54. Balch, James F., M.D., and Phyllis A. Balch, C.N.C,
     Prescription for Nutritional Healing, Garden City Park,
     New York: Avery Publishing Group, 1997, p. 124.

55. Diamond, Harvey and Diamond, Marilyn, *Fit for Life
     II: Living Health -The Complete Health Program,* New
     York: Warner Books, 1987, p. 75.

56. Diamond, Harvey and Diamond, Marilyn, *Fit for Life
     II: Living Health -The Complete Health Program,* New
     York: Warner Books, 1987, p. 75.

57. Weil, Andrew, M.D., *Natural Health, Natural Medi-
     cine*, New York: Houghton Mifflin Company, 1995, p.
     184.

58. Balch, James F., M.D., and Phyllis A. Balch, C.N.C,
     Prescription for Nutritional Healing, Garden City Park,
     New York: Avery Publishing Group, 1997, p. 18.

59. Ginzel, K.H., M.D., "What's in a Cigarette," *ACSH
     Org,* 1997-1998, Available at
     http://www.acsh.org/publications/priorities/0102/nicotin
     e.html. Accessed June 29, 2002.

60. Ginzel, K.H., M.D., "What's in a Cigarette," *ACSH
     Org,* 1997-1998, Available at
     http://www.acsh.org/publications/priorities/0102/nicotin
     e.html. Accessed June 29, 2002.

61.   Ginzel, K.H., M.D., "What's in a Cigarette," *ACSH Org,* 1997-1998, Available at http://www.acsh.org/publications/priorities/0102/nicotine.html. Accessed June 29, 2002.

62.   Carper, Jean, *Food Your Miracle Medicine*, New York: Harper Collins Publishers, 1993, p. 248.

Chapter 12   Drugs vs. Nature – Which is Safer?

1.   "Just How Safe are Herbs?" *Elixir Tonics & Teas*, 1996-2000, Available at http://www.elixir.net/faqs_safety.html. Accessed June 28, 2002.

2.   *Glucosamine and Chondroitin UK Import Ban,* Available at http://www.a1msm.co.uk/017_quality/02_msm_methylsulfonylmethane_to_avoid.htm. Accessed May 29, 2002.

3.   Theodosakis, Jason, M.D., M.S., M.P.H., Brenda Adderly, M.H.A., and Barry Fox, Ph.D., *The Arthritis Cure*, New York: St. Martin's Griffin, 1997, p. 5.

4.   Law, Ron, *Safety of Dietary Supplements*, Available at http://www.laleva.cc/petizione/english/ronlaw_eng.html. Accessed June 28, 2002.

5.   Law, Ron, *Safety of Dietary Supplements*, Available at http://www.laleva.cc/petizione/english/ronlaw_eng.html. Accessed June 28, 2002.

6.   Mercola, Joseph, D.O., *Doctors Are the Third Leading Cause of Death in the U.S., Causing 250,000 Deaths Every Year*, 1997-2002, Available at

http://www.mercola.com/2000/jul/30/doctors_death.htm
. Accessed February 27, 2002.

7.   Staff of University Medical Research, *Amazing Medicines The Drug Companies Don't Want You To Discover*, Tempe, Arizona: University Medical Research Publishers, 1993, p. 20.

8.   Martin, Raquel, and Romano, Karen J., R.N., D.C, *Preventing and Reversing Arthritis Naturally*, Rochester, Vermont: Healing Arts Press, 2000, p. 88-89.

9.   Matsen, John, N.D., *Mysterious Causes and Cures of Illness,* Ohio: Fischer Publishing Corporation, 1995, p. 75-76.

10.   Koehn, Cheryl, Palmer, Tayasha, and Esdaile, John, M.D, *Rheumatoid Arthritis, Plan to Win*, New York: Oxford University Press, 2002, p. 70.

11.   Laux, Marcus, N.D., *Is "Modern" Medicine Killing You?* Potomac, Maryland: Dr. Marcus Laux's Naturally Well, 1995, p. 75.

12.   Weil, Andrew, M.D., *Natural Health, Natural Medicine*, New York: Houghton Mifflin Company, 1995, p. 322.

13.   Martin, Raquel, and Romano, Karen J., R.N., D.C, *Preventing and Reversing Arthritis Naturally*, Rochester, Vermont: Healing Arts Press, 2000, p. 9.

14.   Williams, David G., *Alternatives*, Rockville, Maryland: Mountain Home Publishing, 2002, p. 4.

15.   *Rheumatoid Arthritis Treatments: Learn about the different Arthritis Medications for Treating Arthritis*, 2000-2002, Available at

http://www.allaboutarthritis.com/arthritis.cfm/news/14. html. Accessed February 04, 2002.

16. Airola, Paavo O., N.D., *There is a Cure for Arthritis*, West Nyack, New York: Parker Publishing Company, 1968, p. 36.

17. Matsen, John, N.D., *Mysterious Causes and Cures of Illness,* Ohio: Fischer Publishing Corporation, 1995, p. 70.

18. *Controversial Study Questions Heart Safety of Two Popular Arthritis Drugs*, 2000-2002, Available at http://www.allaboutarthritis.com/arthritis.cfm/news/14. html. Accessed February 04, 2002.

19. Staff of University Medical Research, *Amazing Medicines The Drug Companies Don't Want You To Discover*, Tempe, Arizona: University Medical Research Publishers, 1993, p. 169.

20. Koehn, Cheryl, Palmer, Tayasha, and Esdaile, John, M.D, *Rheumatoid Arthritis, Plan to Win*, New York: Oxford University Press, 2002, p. 70.

21. Lee, Thomas F., Ph.D., *Conquering Rheumatoid Arthritis*, New York: Prometheus Books, 2001, p. 171.

22. Jimenez, Carillo R., M.D., Nurnberger, M., M.D., *Celecoxib-Induced Acute Pancreatitis and Hepatitis: A Case Report*, 1995-2002, Available at http://www.ama-assn.org. Accessed May 17, 2002.

23. Lahita, Robert G., M.D., Ph.D., *Rheumatoid Arthritis-Everything You Need to Know*, New York: Penguin Putnam Inc., 2001, p. 51.

24. Laux, Marcus, N.D., *Is "Modern" Medicine Killing You?* Potomac, Maryland: Dr. Marcus Laux's Naturally Well, 1995, p. 64.

25. Lee, Thomas F., Ph.D., *Conquering Rheumatoid Arthritis*, New York: Prometheus Books, 2001, p. 147.

26. Lee, Thomas F., Ph.D., *Conquering Rheumatoid Arthritis*, New York: Prometheus Books, 2001, p. 146.

27. Lahita, Robert G., M.D., Ph.D., *Rheumatoid Arthritis-Everything You Need to Know*, New York: Penguin Putnam Inc., 2001, p. 58.

28. Mendelson, Robert S., *The People's Doctor, Lets Live*, May 1987, p. 62.

29. Airola, Paavo O., N.D., *There is a Cure for Arthritis*, West Nyack, New York: Parker Publishing Company, 1968, p. 38.

30. Donsbach, Kurt W., D.C., N.D., Ph.D., and Alsleben, H. Rudolph, M.D., D.O., Ph.D., *Arthritis Wholistic Therapy*, Al-Don Institute of Experimental Medicine, 1992, p. 20.

31. Lahita, Robert G., M.D., Ph.D., *Rheumatoid Arthritis - Everything You Need to Know*, New York: Penguin Putnam Inc., 2001, p 50.

32. Pauling, Linus, *How to Live Longer and Feel Better*, New York: W.H. Freeman and Company, 1986, p. 238.

33. Pauling, Linus, *How to Live Longer and Feel Better*, New York: W.H. Freeman and Company, 1986, p. 251.

34. Gaby, Alan, M.D., *Preventing and Reversing Osteoporosis*, Rocklin, California: Prima Publishing, 1994.

35. Nieper, Hans A., M.D., *Biological Approaches to Treatment of Cancer and other Diseases by Hans Nieper,* 1997-2000, Available at http://www.heall.com/healingnews/july/nieper.html. Accessed May 28, 2002.

Chapter 13 Health vs. Wealth – The Money Factor

1. Pauling, Linus, *How to Live Longer and Feel Better*, New York: W.H. Freeman and Company, 1986, p. 251.

2. Theodosakis, Jason, M.D., M.S., M.P.H., Brenda Adderly, M.H.A., and Barry Fox, Ph.D. *The Arthritis Cure.* New York: St. Martin's Griffin, 1997, p.50.

3. Laux, Marcus, N.D. *Is "Modern" Medicine Killing You?* Potomac, Maryland: Dr. Marcus Laux's Naturally Well, 1995, p. 10.

4. Laux, Marcus, N.D., *Is "Modern" Medicine Killing You?* Potomac, Maryland: Dr. Marcus Laux's Naturally Well, 1995, p. 49.

5. Gaby, Alan, M.D., *Preventing and Reversing Osteoporosis*, Rocklin, California: Prima Publishing, 1994, p30.

6. Airola, Paavo O., N.D., *There is a Cure for Arthritis*, West Nyack, New York: Parker Publishing Company, 1968, p. 20.

7. Airola, Paavo O., N.D., *There is a Cure for Arthritis*, West Nyack, New York: Parker Publishing Company, 1968, p. 20.

8. Staff of University Medical Research, *Amazing Medicines The Drug Companies Don't Want You To Dis-*

cover, Tempe, Arizona: University Medical Research Publishers, 1993, p. 33.

9.   Irving Levin Associates, *Health Care Executive Compensation Report 2001*, Available at http://www.levinassociates.com. Accessed June 29, 2002.

10. Diamond, Harvey and Diamond, Marilyn, *Fit for Life II: Living Health -The Complete Health Program,* New York: Warner Books, 1987, p. 76.

11. Laux, Marcus, N.D., *Is "Modern" Medicine Killing You?* Potomac, Maryland: Dr. Marcus Laux's Naturally Well, 1995, p. 72.

12. Staff of University Medical Research, *Amazing Medicines The Drug Companies Don't Want You To Discover*, Tempe, Arizona: University Medical Research Publishers, 1993, p. 4.

13. Theodosakis, Jason, M.D., M.S., M.P.H., Brenda Adderly, M.H.A., and Barry Fox, Ph.D. *The Arthritis Cure*. New York: St. Martin's Griffin, 1997, p.50.

14. Lawrence, Ronald, "Inflammatory Drugs for Aching Joints Could Send You to the Hospital," *Journal of Longevity* 4, no. 6, 1998, p. 21.

15. Holland, Eileen G., PHARM.D., and Degruy, Frank V., M.D., *American Family Physician-Drug-Induced Disorders,* 1997, Available at http://www.aafp.org/afp/971101ap/holland.html. Accessed February 27, 2002.

16. Murray, Michael T., N.D., *Natural Alternatives to Over-the-Counter and Prescription Drugs*, New York: William Morrow and Company Inc., 1994, p. 21.

17. Staff of University Medical Research, *Amazing Medicines The Drug Companies Don't Want You To Discover*, Tempe, Arizona: University Medical Research Publishers, 1993, p. 24.

18. Laux, Marcus, N.D., *Is "Modern" Medicine Killing You?* Potomac, Maryland: Dr. Marcus Laux's Naturally Well, 1995, p. 72.

19. Mercola, Joseph, D.O., *Medical Mistakes Kill 100,000 Americans a Year*, 1997-2002, Available at http://www.mercola.com/1999/dec/5/medical_mistakes.html. Accessed February 27, 2002.

20. Ashby, Cheryl, C.C.T., "Problems Associated with Colon Toxicity," *The Colon Health Network*, 1997-2002, Available at http://colonhealth.net. Accessed June 04, 2002.

21. Lee, Thomas F., Ph.D., *Conquering Rheumatoid Arthritis*, New York: Prometheus Books, 2001, p. 169.

22. Staff of University Medical Research, *Amazing Medicines The Drug Companies Don't Want You To Discover*, Tempe, Arizona: University Medical Research Publishers, 1993, p. 10.

23. Matsen, John, N.D., *Mysterious Causes and Cures of Illness,* Ohio: Fischer Publishing Corporation, 1995, p. 70.

24. Null, Gary, Ph.D., *Gary Null's Ultimate Lifetime Diet*, New York: Broadway Books, 2000, p. 159.

25. Mercola, Joseph, D.O., *Doctors Are the Third Leading Cause of Death in the U.S., Causing 250,000 Deaths Every Year*, 1997-2002, Available at

http://www.mercola.com/2000/jul/30/doctors_death.ht
m. Accessed February 27, 2002.

26. Mercola, Joseph, D.O., *Doctors Are the Third Leading Cause of Death in the U.S., Causing 250,000 Deaths Every Year*, 1997-2002, Available at http://www.mercola.com/2000/jul/30/doctors_death.ht m. Accessed February 27, 2002.

27. Murray, Michael T., N.D., *Natural Alternatives to Over-the-Counter and Prescription Drugs*, New York: William Morrow and Company Inc., 1994, p. 22.

28. Mercola, Joseph, D.O., *Doctors Are the Third Leading Cause of Death in the U.S., Causing 250,000 Deaths Every Year*, 1997-2002, Available at http://www.mercola.com/2000/jul/30/doctors_death.ht m. Accessed February 27, 2002.

29. Matsen, John, N.D., *Mysterious Causes and Cures of Illness,* Ohio: Fischer Publishing Corporation, 1995, p. 142.

30. *Leading Causes of Death*, Available at http://lifematters.com/deathcaus.html. Accessed February 27, 2002.

31. Matsen, John, N.D., *Mysterious Causes and Cures of Illness,* Ohio: Fischer Publishing Corporation, 1995, p. 140.

32. Null, Gary, Ph.D., *Gary Null's Ultimate Lifetime Diet*, New York: Broadway Books, 2000, p. 144.

33. Staff of University Medical Research, *Amazing Medicines The Drug Companies Don't Want You To Discover*, Tempe, Arizona: University Medical Research Publishers, 1993, p. 41.

34. Laux, Marcus, N.D., *Is "Modern" Medicine Killing You?* Potomac, Maryland: Dr. Marcus Laux's Naturally Well, 1995, p. 52.

35. *Arthritis, Your Orthopedic Connection-American Academy of Orthopedic Surgeons*, 1995-2001, Available at http://orthoinfo.aaos.org. Accessed February 2, 2002.

36. *Arthritis by the Numbers, All About Arthritis*, 2000-2002, Available at http://www.allaboutarthritis.com. Accessed February 19, 2002.

37. *Arthritis, Your Orthopedic Connection-American Academy of Orthopedic Surgeons*, 1995-2001, Available at http://orthoinfo.aaos.org. Accessed February 2, 2002.

38. *Arthritis by the Numbers, All About Arthritis*, 2000-2002, Available at http://www.allaboutarthritis.com. Accessed February 19, 2002.

Bibliography

Airola, Paavo O., N.D. *There is a Cure for Arthritis.* West Nyack, New York: Parker Publishing Company, 1968.

Ali, Majid, M.D. *The Ghoraa and Limbic Exercise.* Denville, New Jersey: IPM Press, 1993.

Balch, James F., M.D., and Phyllis A. Balch, C.N.C. *Prescription for Nutritional Healing.* Garden City Park, New York: Avery Publishing Group, 1997.

Burton Goldberg Group. *Alternative Medicine: The Definitive Guide.* Washington: Future Medicine Publishing, 1993.

Cameron, Ewan, and Pauling, Linus. *Cancer and Vitamin C.* Menlo Park, California: Linus Pauling Institute of Science and Medicine, 1979.

Carper, Jean. *Food Your Miracle Medicine.* New York: Harper Collins Publishers, 1993.

Chopra, Deepak, M.D. *Ageless Body Timeless Mind.* New York: Harmony Books, 1993.

Cousins, Norman. *Anatomy of an Illness As Perceived by the Patient.* New York: W.W. Norton & Company, 1979.

Diamond, Harvey and Marilyn Diamond. *Fit for Life.* New York: Warner Books, 1985.

Diamond, Harvey and Marilyn Diamond. *Fit for Life II: Living Health -The Complete Health Program.* New York: Warner Books, 1987.

Donsbach, Kurt W., D.C., N.D., Ph.D., and Alsleben, H. Rudolph, M.D., D.O., Ph.D. *Arthritis Wholistic Therapy.* Al-Don Institute of Experimental Medicine, 1992.

Eisenstein, Phyllis, and Scheiner, Samuel M., Ph.D. *Overcoming the Pain of Inflammatory Arthritis.* Garden City Park, New York: Avery Publishing Group, 1997.

Fox, Barry, Ph.D. *Arthritis for Dummies.* New York: Hungry Minds, Inc., 2000.

Fries, James F., M.D. *Arthritis: A Take Care of Yourself Help Guide.* Cambridge, Massachusetts: Perseus Books, 1994.

Gerson, Max, M.D. *A Cancer Therapy-Results of Fifty Cases.* Barrytown, New York: Station Hill Press, 1997.

Hass, Elson M., M.D. *Staying Healthy with Nutrition.* Berkeley, California: Celestial Arts, 1992.

Henry, Sara J. *John Hopkins Health, Arthritis: What You Need to Know.* Alexandria, Virginia: Time Life Books, 1999.

Horne, Steven H. *Constitutional Iridology.* Provo, Utah: Tree of Light Institute, Inc., 1997.

Horstman, Judith. *The Arthritis Foundation's Guide to Alternative Therapies.* Atlanta, Georgia: The Arthritis Foundation, 1999.

Ivker, Robert S., D.O., and Nelson, Todd, N.D. *Arthritis Survival, The Holistic Medical Treatment Program for Osteoarthritis.* New York: Penguin Putnam, Inc., 2001.

Jarvis, D.C., M.D. *Arthritis and Folk Medicine*. New York: Fawcett Crest, 1960.

Jensen, Bernard, Ph.D. *Juicing Therapy*. Los Angeles, California: Keats Publishing, 2000.

Koehn, Cheryl, Palmer, Tayasha, and Esdaile, John, M.D. *Rheumatoid Arthritis, Plan to Win*. New York: Oxford University Press, 2002.

Lahita, Robert G., M.D., Ph.D. *Rheumatoid Arthritis- Everything You Need to Know*. New York: Penguin Putnam Inc., 2001.

Lane, Nancy E., M.D., and Wallace, Danielle J., M.D. *All About Osteoarthritis, The Definitive Resource for Arthritis Patients and their Families*. New York: Oxford University Press, 2002.

Laux, Marcus, N.D. *Is "Modern" Medicine Killing You?* Potomac, Maryland: Dr. Marcus Laux's Naturally Well, 1995.

Lee, Thomas F., Ph.D. *Conquering Rheumatoid Arthritis*. New York: Promethus Books, 2001.

Mae, Eydie, and Loeffler, Chris. *How I Conquered Cancer Naturally*. Garden City Park, New York: Avery Publishing Group, 1992.

Margen, Sheldon, M.D., and the Editors of the University of California at Berkeley Wellness Letter. *The Wellness Encyclopedia of Food and Nutrition*. New York: Random House, 1992.

Martin, Raquel, and Romano, Karen J., R.N., D.C. *Preventing and Reversing Arthritis Naturally*. Rochester, Vermont: Healing Arts Press, 2000.

Matsen, John, N.D. *Mysterious Causes and Cures of Illness.* Canfield, Ohio: Fischer Publishing Corporation, 1995.

Mindell, Earl, R.Ph., Ph.D. *Earl Mindell's Food as Medicine.* New York: Simon & Schuster, 1994.

Murray, Michael T., N.D. *Natural Alternatives to Over-the-Counter and Prescription Drugs.* New York: William Morrow and Company Inc., 1994.

Null, Gary, Ph.D. *Gary Null's Ultimate Lifetime Diet.* New York: Broadway Books, 2000.

Pauling, Linus, Ph.D. *How to Live Longer and Feel Better.* New York: W.H. Freeman and Company, 1986.

Sobel, Dava, and Klein, Arthur C. *Arthritis: What Works.* New York: St. Martin Press, 1989.

Staff of University Medical Research. *Amazing Medicines The Drug Companies Don't Want You To Discover.* Tempe, Arizona: University Medical Research Publishers, 1993.

Theodosakis, Jason, M.D., M.S., M.P.H., Brenda Adderly, M.H.A., and Barry Fox, Ph.D. *The Arthritis Cure.* New York: St. Martin's Griffin, 1997.

Ulman, Dana. *Homeopathy Medicine for the 21st Century.* Berkeley, California: North Atlantic Books, 1988.

Wade, Carlson. *Inner Cleansing- How to Free Yourself From Joint-Muscle-Artery-Circulation Sludge.* West Nyack, New York: Parker Publishing Company, 1992.

Weil, Andrew, M.D. *Eating Well for Optimum Health.* New York: Alfred A. Knopf, 2000.

Weil, Andrew, M.D. *Natural Health, Natural Medicine*. New York: Houghton Mifflin Company, 1995.

Welsh, Philip J., D.D.S., N.D., and Leonardo, Bianca, N.D. *Freedom From Arthritis Through Nutrition*. Joshua Tree, California: Tree of Life Publication, 1992.

Zampieron, Eugene R., N.D., A.H.G., and Kamhi, Ellen, R.N., H.N.C. *Arthritis: An Alternative Medicine Definitive Guide*. Tiburon, California: AlternativeMedicine.com, 1999.

Index

acidophilus 85, 95
Acidophilus 94, 245, 255
additives ... 95, 153, 192, 195
adrenal glands 81
advil 105
Advil 15, 18
Albert Schweitzer 33
alcohol16, 37, 43, 44, 52, 55,
    69, 70, 95, 98, 150, 154,
    176, 182, 186
alfalfa 62, 85
Alfalfa 62
alkaline foods 39
allergies 49, 65, 206, 221
alpha-lipoic acid 95, 96
aluminum 133, 192
Alzheimer's disease 192
American Holistic Medical
    Association 69
amino acid 105
animals 37, 162, 167
ankle .. 18, 21, 25, 41, 51, 56,
    89, 97
Ankylosing Spondylitis .. 22,
    26, 47, 115
antibiotics .. 60, 66, 125, 128,
    188, 189, 212, 213, 223
antibodies 53, 190
anticancer 162

anti-inflammatory 42, 65, 67,
    96, 97, 100, 102, 120,
    165, 210, 211
antioxidant 68, 69, 95, 96,
    106, 112, 113, 221
antioxidants . 65, 95, 96, 106,
    131, 159, 190, 219
appetite 64, 67, 129
apple cider vinegar 97
applied kinesiologist 59
arachidonic acid 39, 167
arteries 39, 114, 160
arteriosclerosis 65, 151
arthritis 7, 8, 9, 11, 12, 21,
    22, 23, 24, 25, 26, 27, 28,
    29, 30, 34, 35, 37, 39, 40,
    44, 45, 46, 47, 51, 52, 53,
    56, 57, 60, 61, 62, 64, 65,
    67, 68, 70, 71, 72, 74, 77,
    79, 87, 89, 91, 92, 96, 97,
    98, 100, 102, 105, 106,
    107, 108, 109, 110, 117,
    120, 122, 124, 125, 126,
    128, 132, 135, 137, 141,
    144, 145, 146, 147, 148,
    151, 152, 154, 157, 158,
    160, 167, 169, 170, 198,
    200, 210, 212, 213, 214,
    216, 217, 219, 225, 226,
    229, 265, 266

artificial colors 94, 174
aspartame 186
aspirin ... 47, 67, 70, 71, 111,
    128, 192, 210, 211, 212,
    213, 214
asthma 28, 96, 154, 160
atherosclerosis........ 113, 160
autoimmune .. 12, 22, 30, 34,
    91, 98, 102, 145
bacteria.... 43, 46, 47, 53, 66,
    94, 133, 135, 212
Beans................................ 38
bile 67, 122
bioflavonoid................... 106
bioflavonoids 112, 124
blood . 11, 18, 20, 22, 26, 27,
    28, 41, 42, 43, 46, 48, 51,
    52, 53, 63, 65, 66, 67, 68,
    71, 72, 74, 75, 77, 78, 79,
    93, 97, 98, 100, 102, 104,
    106, 110, 112, 114, 122,
    124, 127, 128, 129, 130,
    131, 135, 143, 152, 167,
    168, 184, 196, 197, 200,
    211, 212, 217, 225
Blood Circulation............. 59
blood clots...................... 100
blood plasma.................... 78
blood pressure110, 112, 168,
    197
blood stream............... 71, 78
blood vessels... 77, 110, 167,
    197
bloodstream... 48, 50, 52, 61,
    68, 78, 140, 141, 197
body 8, 9, 11, 16, 17, 18, 20,
    21, 22, 23, 24, 27, 28, 30,
    31, 34, 35, 38, 39, 40, 41,

42, 43, 44, 46, 47, 48, 49,
    50, 51, 52, 55, 58, 59, 60,
    61, 62, 64, 67, 68, 70, 71,
    73, 76, 77, 78, 79, 80, 81,
    82, 83, 86, 87, 88, 89, 90,
    93, 94, 95, 96, 97, 100,
    103, 104, 106, 107, 108,
    109, 110, 111, 112, 114,
    115, 119, 120, 121, 122,
    123, 124, 125, 126, 127,
    128, 129, 130, 131, 132,
    134, 135, 136, 137, 139,
    140, 141, 142, 143, 144,
    145, 146, 147, 150, 154,
    155, 157, 158, 159, 160,
    162, 163, 165, 166, 169,
    170, 171, 172, 173, 175,
    176, 177, 181, 182, 183,
    184, 186, 188, 190, 191,
    192, 193, 196, 197, 198,
    200, 202, 214, 215, 216,
    218, 229, 231
bromelain 85, 97, 98, 246
brown rice 158, 163, 164
Brown Rice 38
bursitis...................... 97, 120
butter 158, 159, 162, 164,
    165, 173, 181, 182
caffeine..... 44, 121, 150, 186
Caffeine........................... 76
calcium...... 62, 94, 134, 159,
    160, 172, 183, 188, 214
cancer 27, 35, 37, 65, 69, 93,
    100, 113, 118, 128, 151,
    152, 154, 157, 161, 164,
    170, 182, 185, 186, 193,
    194, 195, 196, 200, 217,
    223, 224, 232

Cancer. 27, 36, 69, 109, 138, 207, 232, 251, 267, 273, 274, 276
candida 75
candidiasis 95
canned 38, 40, 154
capsules 36, 94, 104, 114
carbohydrate . 163, 169, 170, 177
carbohydrates .. 63, 104, 140, 142, 169, 185
carbon dioxide 130, 131, 143
cardiovascular .. 66, 67, 113, 143, 212
cardiovascular system 67
carpal tunnel syndrome .. 120
cartilage. 100, 104, 105, 124, 144, 145
castor oil 117, 118, 120
cayenne ... 63, 122, 237, 238, 242
Cayenne 62, 63, 121, 237, 242
Celebrex 212
Celecoxib 213, 266
cell11, 40, 58, 65, 75, 76, 77, 78, 81, 106, 130, 143, 167, 171, 182
cells ... 40, 43, 44, 49, 52, 65, 68, 73, 75, 76, 77, 79, 97, 105, 109, 120, 121, 124, 127, 129, 130, 131, 132, 135, 143, 152, 162, 167, 171, 186, 189, 190, 196, 197
Chapman University .. 14, 23
cherry juice 98
Chicken 38

Chiropractic 10, 58, 241
chiropractic adjustments .. 58
chiropractor ... 17, 18, 25, 26, 30, 33, 143
cholesterol62, 63, 66, 67, 72, 112, 114, 164, 165, 168, 184, 211
chondroitin sulfate . 104, 219
Chronic Conditions 88
chronic disease 78
chronic fatigue 47
chronic liver inflammation 96
cigarette. 185, 194, 195, 196, 197, 198
circulation . 53, 67, 107, 117, 120, 123, 192
cirrhosis 69
cod liver oil 100, 101
coffee. 47, 56, 117, 119, 150, 154
colic 161
collagen .. 105, 106, 112, 124
colon .. 41, 45, 46, 48, 50, 72, 83, 108, 117, 118, 119, 162, 185, 223
Colon Cleanse 85
Colon cleansing 46
common cold 63, 88, 223
connective tissue 78, 106
cortisone 211, 212, 214
crippling 7, 9, 24, 148
CYCLE
DETOXIFICATION 83
d-alpha tocopherol 113
death rate 69, 93, 225
deaths 10, 133, 204, 209, 210, 211, 213, 224

deformed 9, 34, 127, 148
degenerative .. 27, 35, 37, 48,
  64, 76, 93, 103, 109, 113,
  120, 126, 128, 151, 152,
  154, 157, 188, 218
detoxification .. 8, 27, 28, 35,
  40, 41, 43, 45, 48, 50, 52,
  69, 71, 73, 83, 104, 121,
  123, 139, 143, 233, 235,
  236, 239, 251, 255, 262
detoxify 43, 49, 83, 131, 143
DETOXIFYING BATH 119
Devil's claw 63
diabetes 28, 35, 93, 128, 151,
  154
diagnosis ... 8, 23, 24, 25, 26,
  31, 75
diagnostic tests 59
diarrhea ... 43, 124, 129, 206,
  213
diet 11, 39, 44, 76, 78, 93,
  98, 103, 109, 110, 140,
  149, 150, 152, 154, 157,
  159, 160, 161, 164, 166,
  168, 169, 170, 171, 181,
  186, 229
digestion .. 50, 76, 78, 79, 81,
  97, 103, 104, 122, 129,
  135, 136, 137, 139, 140,
  141, 142, 151, 170, 184
Digestive 35, 36, 59, 136,
  248
digestive system 49, 159
digestive tract 71, 94, 184
disease 7, 8, 9, 10, 24, 25, 27,
  28, 29, 30, 34, 35, 39, 42,
  44, 47, 48, 52, 53, 56, 59,
  60, 65, 70, 75, 77, 78, 81,
  88, 90, 93, 96, 98, 100,
  102, 103, 108, 112, 113,
  115, 122, 126, 127, 128,
  129, 137, 142, 145, 146,
  147, 149, 150, 151, 152,
  153, 155, 157, 158, 159,
  167, 168, 170, 171, 184,
  185, 189, 191, 192, 194,
  197, 198, 212, 213, 223,
  224, 230, 249
diseases 7, 28, 35, 37, 44, 65,
  67, 76, 79, 88, 93, 110,
  113, 128, 136, 151, 152,
  157, 188, 225
distilled water. 119, 122, 135
Distilled water 135
Distilled Water 121, 122
DMSO 102, 120, 247
doctor 4, 7, 8, 10, 17, 19, 20,
  21, 23, 24, 25, 27, 29, 30,
  31, 51, 56, 57, 59, 82, 86,
  87, 115, 149, 201, 204,
  206, 213, 217, 218, 219,
  220, 230
doctors ... 7, 8, 11, 17, 20, 21,
  24, 40, 41, 47, 57, 58, 66,
  75, 86, 89, 92, 102, 108,
  176, 199, 200, 201, 204,
  208, 210, 214, 217, 218,
  220, 222, 223, 225, 226,
  231, 250, 264, 270, 271
drug . 8, 9, 10, 38, 58, 64, 66,
  70, 105, 126, 194, 198,
  199, 200, 204, 206, 208,
  211, 212, 217, 220, 221,
  222
drugs 7, 8, 29, 41, 44, 52, 55,
  58, 60, 61, 66, 68, 75, 88,

95, 108, 111, 127, 128,
146, 153, 199, 200, 201,
203, 204, 206, 207, 208,
210, 211, 212, 213, 214,
217, 218, 220, 221, 229,
230
dry heat sauna 51, 53
education... 11, 64, 200, 219,
224, 238
Eggs 38, 181
elastin 106
enemas 46, 47, 118, 119
Enemas 36, 45, 46
Enriched foods 162
enzymes 49, 50, 63, 95, 103,
104, 105, 137, 139, 140,
256
Enzymes 35, 36, 50, 103,
136, 139, 247, 248, 256,
258
esophagus 182
exercise 11, 51, 53, 122, 127,
130, 142, 143, 144, 150,
154, 155
eyes ... 27, 33, 53, 61, 75, 78,
80, 103, 112, 128, 130,
208
fat free foods 149
fats... 44, 137, 152, 159, 164,
165, 166, 167, 168, 182,
183, 184
fatty acids 100, 161, 165,
167, 183, 184
Federal Drug Administration
.... 204, 205
fever 52, 70, 71, 129
Fever 43
Feverfew 64, 65, 238

fiber 85, 94, 163, 169
Fish 38
flavonol 65
flu 66, 74, 88, 128, 213
fluoride 133, 134
food8, 37, 39, 41, 43, 44, 46,
48, 89, 92, 93, 95, 98,
103, 104, 109, 113, 123,
136, 137, 139, 140, 141,
142, 149, 150, 152, 153,
154, 157, 158, 159, 160,
162, 163, 165, 166, 169,
171, 174, 176, 177, 181,
183, 185, 188, 189, 190,
192, 202, 225, 230
Food and Drug
Administration 64
FOOD ENZYMES 102
formaldehyde 131, 186
free radicals. 68, 69, 96, 106,
112
gall bladder 122, 123
garlic . 65, 66, 123, 171, 172,
219
Garlic 65, 66, 123, 239
gastrointestinal tract . 94, 140
Gelotology 147
Geneticists 11
German Commission E ... 63,
69
germs 200
Gerson27, 28, 31, 33, 34, 35,
36, 37, 38, 39, 41, 45, 47,
48, 49, 50, 51, 54, 57, 73,
75, 232, 233, 235, 262,
274
Ginger 67, 119, 123, 239,
240

Glucosamine .. 104, 248, 264
gout 98
Grape seed extract.......... 106
HDL 112, 164, 168
headache 46, 64, 206
headaches.... 64, 65, 71, 132, 197, 206
healing27, 33, 35, 42, 45, 50, 52, 55, 56, 58, 65, 70, 71, 74, 78, 82, 88, 90, 93, 102, 112, 117, 124, 129, 137, 147, 148, 158, 188, 229
healing crisis 74
healing environment 27, 229
health... 8, 10, 11, 12, 16, 27, 28, 45, 46, 48, 51, 52, 53, 57, 58, 59, 61, 62, 66, 68, 71, 74, 75, 77, 78, 79, 80, 82, 87, 89, 90, 91, 92, 93, 96, 97, 109, 110, 111, 122, 123, 124, 126, 127, 129, 132, 133, 134, 135, 137, 139, 140, 144, 145, 150, 152, 154, 155, 157, 158, 160, 162, 164, 166, 170, 171, 176, 178, 180, 181, 183, 185, 186, 188, 191, 192, 193, 198, 200, 201, 202, 203, 204, 210, 214, 217, 219, 220, 223, 224, 225, 227, 228, 231, 238, 246
health conditions.............. 92
heart attack 63, 71, 100, 151, 165, 194, 212
heart attacks 110, 168
heart conditions.............. 114

heart disease...... 53, 93, 151, 152, 185, 225
hemoglobin 97
herbology . 56, 60, 61, 62, 73
herbs.... 8, 60, 61, 62, 64, 65, 73, 82, 96, 199, 200, 202, 204, 215, 219, 221, 237, 241, 248
high blood pressure... 11, 27, 28, 93, 110, 128, 152, 168, 184, 200, 212, 217
high cholesterol. 11, 62, 128, 200, 217
high fructose corn syrup 172, 174
Hippocrates 37, 46, 137, 199
hips....................... 18, 20, 85
histamine................ 106, 111
HLA-B27 22
holistic............................. 28
homeopathic remedy........ 89
homeopathy.......... 87, 88, 91
Honey............... 38, 121, 146
hospital..... 21, 208, 222, 231
Hubbard Purification Program................... 51, 53
hyaluronan..................... 105
hydrogenated. 159, 165, 166, 173, 181, 182, 183
hypertension............. 46, 110
iatrogenic...................... 210
ibuprofen...................... 105
immune system 8, 11, 27, 28, 35, 40, 41, 42, 43, 46, 49, 70, 75, 79, 102, 103, 108, 111, 121, 126, 127, 128, 129, 130, 140, 143, 145,

150, 152, 154, 159, 181, 182, 190, 201, 225

incurable 8, 9, 12, 22, 23, 24, 25, 28, 29, 56, 146, 229

inflammation. 22, 26, 39, 41, 42, 43, 46, 51, 53, 64, 70, 71, 79, 96, 97, 98, 107, 117, 120, 165, 167, 186

intestinal flora 95

iodine 107, 159, 188

Iodine 35, 36, 107, 156

Iridology 79, 80, 243, 275

iris 79, 80, 81

IRIS ANALYSIS 79

joint... 14, 21, 30, 34, 43, 64, 67, 97, 100, 105, 120, 125, 144, 148, 213

joints ... 9, 11, 18, 20, 22, 29, 30, 34, 42, 47, 64, 67, 72, 97, 102, 104, 105, 106, 118, 121, 124, 126, 127, 137, 144, 145, 154, 160, 170, 211

Journal of American College of Cardiology 53

juicing . 8, 28, 36, 48, 49, 50, 73, 79, 104

Karen Romano 38, 105, 127, 132

Kelp........................... 36, 107

Kidney Cleanse 85

kidney failure 211

kidneys.. 41, 43, 52, 81, 118, 121, 122, 128, 135, 197, 213

kinesiology.... 56, 59, 60, 61, 73, 82

large intestine 46

law of similars 88

laxative 44

LDL 62, 113, 114, 164

liquids 41, 68, 137

LIVE CELL ANALYSIS. 74

liver ... 36, 41, 43, 46, 48, 68, 69, 75, 78, 96, 100, 117, 118, 121, 122, 123, 128, 143, 162, 176, 182, 192, 201, 212

Liver Cleanse 85

Long-term health............ 176

lower back 17, 18, 25, 64, 90, 118

lungs.. 41, 43, 129, 131, 135, 143, 197, 198

Marcus Ettinger.... 3, 33, 232

margarine 158, 159, 162, 165, 181, 183, 230

Max Gerson... 27, 28, 30, 33, 35, 57, 107, 109

medical 4, 7, 8, 9, 12, 24, 29, 30, 31, 38, 39, 53, 58, 60, 66, 67, 71, 82, 87, 92, 111, 128, 176, 192, 200, 202, 205, 207, 217, 218, 219, 220, 221, 223, 224, 231, 232, 270

medical system 200

medication. 4, 15, 22, 23, 24, 25, 26, 28, 29, 30, 31, 40, 41, 42, 45, 47, 55, 67, 126, 127, 206, 210, 211, 212, 217

medications . 4, 7, 10, 25, 29, 31, 41, 42, 67, 118, 127, 200, 204, 214, 217, 230

medicine 7, 9, 33, 37, 42, 57, 60, 63, 67, 69, 70, 76, 87, 88, 89, 90, 91, 102, 118, 128, 129, 145, 146, 149, 199, 201, 206, 212, 214, 218, 219, 223, 230
metabolic support............. 75
metabolism.... 11, 53, 78, 94, 107
methods... 8, 37, 45, 58, 189, 200, 217, 220
migraine 65, 71
migraines........................ 28
milk 68, 69, 85, 94, 117, 159, 160, 161, 162, 182, 183, 190
Milk thistle................. 68, 69
minerals... 39, 49, 62, 93, 94, 103, 107, 135, 155, 162, 163, 186, 188, 221, 252
monounsaturated fat164, 168
Monounsaturated fat 164
MSM..... 108, 109, 219, 247, 250
mucous membranes 106
multiple sclerosis 35
MULTIVITAMIN 93
murders 211
muscles . 11, 15, 59, 78, 102, 137, 145
mustard 171, 172, 178
Naprosyn........................ 22
natural ... 8, 9, 27, 28, 29, 30, 31, 33, 34, 37, 38, 40, 42, 45, 46, 50, 52, 55, 56, 58, 60, 62, 65, 66, 67, 69, 71, 73, 74, 75, 76, 79, 80, 82, 86, 88, 89, 92, 96, 98, 100, 102, 109, 112, 115, 117, 122, 123, 125, 126, 136, 146, 147, 148, 154, 157, 158, 162, 163, 170, 171, 172, 173, 174, 175, 176, 180, 183, 184, 189, 191, 192, 200, 215, 217, 220, 221, 229, 231
natural foods....... 55, 73, 157
natural programs 56, 74, 231
nerves 17
Niacin.................... 35, 156
niacinamide 85
Non Toxic 89
nontoxic........................... 88
NSAID's211, 212, 213, 214, 223
nutrients... 35, 42, 44, 46, 48, 49, 50, 74, 78, 94, 96, 103, 105, 107, 109, 121, 132, 143, 144, 147, 154, 157
nutrition8, 11, 27, 37, 56, 68, 94, 103, 113, 144, 146, 150, 152, 166, 205, 218, 219, 252
nutritional deficiencies..... 75
Oatmeal........................... 38
ODA....... 154, 155, 156, 157
Olestra........................... 184
olive oil . 120, 123, 164, 166, 168, 181
Omega-3......... 100, 161, 165
Omega-6.............. 165, 167
OPC's........................... 106
optometry 112
organic... 28, 35, 38, 97, 107, 119, 188, 189

organic foods ... 28, 188, 189
organs 43, 49, 59, 61, 82, 83, 143, 214
orthopedic doctor 21, 25
osteoarthritis 34, 64, 68, 105, 112, 213, 238
osteopathic physician 87
osteoporosis 11, 39, 93, 134, 151
oxidative damage 114
oxygen... 102, 121, 129, 130, 131, 132, 143, 146, 147, 196
oxygenation...................... 76
pain . 7, 9, 14, 15, 16, 17, 18, 20, 21, 22, 24, 25, 26, 28, 29, 30, 37, 43, 47, 48, 53, 55, 60, 63, 64, 67, 68, 70, 71, 72, 73, 89, 90, 99, 100, 102, 105, 107, 108, 109, 117, 118, 119, 120, 121, 125, 126, 127, 129, 132, 144, 145, 147, 148, 193, 201, 206, 213, 221, 229
painkillers 42
pantothenic acid 85
parasites 46, 75, 133
patented drug 221
patient . 7, 17, 29, 31, 33, 44, 57, 64, 70, 89, 90, 91, 204, 210, 214, 217
peanut butter 173
Peanut Butter ... 38, 172, 173
pesticides.. 68, 133, 188, 189
pharmaceutical companies 205, 208, 217, 220
pharmacies 70

phosphorous 160
phytochemicals 49
placebo 64, 69, 106
plantar fasciitis 15
plants 37, 61, 131, 188
polyunsaturated 159, 165, 166, 167
potassium 39, 40, 62, 109, 110, 163, 171, 183, 189
Potassium ... 35, 36, 156, 250
Potatoes 38
prescribed.. 7, 25, 26, 36, 37, 42, 71, 90, 199, 205, 206, 207, 211, 212, 213
prescription ... 4, 8, 9, 22, 60, 66, 127, 153, 199, 201, 203, 204, 211, 217
preservatives 95, 153
probiotics......................... 94
professionals 7, 8, 231
programs 8, 9, 27, 31, 40, 51, 56, 57, 60, 61, 73, 74, 75, 79, 82, 86, 87, 88, 89, 90, 92, 115, 117, 118, 125, 127, 146, 147, 148, 205, 217, 220, 221, 228, 229, 230
prostaglandins 39, 67, 70, 96
protease inhibitors 162
protein 39, 68, 104, 137, 140, 141, 142, 160, 169, 185
proteins..... 44, 104, 141, 182
proteoglycans 105
psoriasis.......................... 96
putrefaction 140
Ralph Moss 40
Raquel Martin . 38, 105, 127, 132

RDA111, 154, 155, 156, 157

red blood cells76, 77, 79, 97, 127, 196

Reiter's Syndrome 22, 26, 47, 115

research. 8, 9, 11, 25, 28, 29, 61, 64, 71, 72, 87, 92, 97, 100, 103, 104, 105, 114, 115, 147, 190, 192, 219, 231, 249

responsible .. 10, 12, 78, 114, 151, 204

retina 103, 107, 213

reverse osmosis.............. 135

rheumatic conditions64, 226, 227

rheumatoid 21, 34, 67, 68, 102, 108, 213

rheumatoid arthritis. 34, 102, 108

rheumatologist 21, 25, 26, 27, 28, 29, 30, 31

riboflavin.................. 85, 163

Rye Bread 38

salicylic acid 70

salt. 111, 119, 171, 172, 173, 174, 182, 183

saponin............................ 71

Saturated fat.................... 164

sauna program...... 52, 53, 54

school...... 8, 14, 23, 31, 153, 200, 218, 219, 220

sedative 44

selenium.................. 159, 189

seronegative polyarthritis. 34

seropositve polyarthritis... 34

side effects 30, 44, 59, 67, 70, 72, 88, 106, 118, 204, 206, 211, 213, 214, 221

sinusitis 98

skin.... 18, 28, 47, 49, 51, 52, 53, 89, 106, 107, 119, 120, 123, 124, 143, 164, 191, 192

Skin brushing 123

skin diseases..................... 28

skin disorders 47, 49

sleep 21, 44, 47, 130, 134, 145, 146, 150, 216

smokers ... 76, 193, 194, 196, 197

smoking. 127, 154, 185, 193, 194, 198

sodium..... 39, 109, 110, 134, 171, 172, 174, 183, 189, 191

soy 94, 161, 182, 183

Soy Milk........... 38, 159, 161

spinal cord....................... 58

spine 18, 22, 29, 58

standard American diet .. 154

Stephen T. Sinatra............ 39

stomach ... 29, 41, 43, 63, 67, 70, 78, 95, 97, 104, 117, 124, 128, 132, 136, 137, 138, 141, 161, 182, 206, 211, 212, 214

stomach pains........... 29, 136

Stop 7, 193

strength training............. 143

stroke... 27, 65, 71, 100, 110, 113, 170, 252

strokes 39, 110, 184, 200, 225

suffering 9, 91, 98, 109, 204, 221, 229

sugar 98, 104, 111, 117, 152, 154, 172, 173, 174, 177, 180, 182, 183, 184, 186

supplements .. 35, 66, 71, 79, 83, 92, 93, 94, 95, 96, 103, 104, 105, 106, 107, 108, 118, 125, 202, 205, 206, 207, 215, 221, 222

surgeries.. 10, 126, 200, 217, 225

surgery 7, 31, 127, 210, 218, 221, 222, 225

sweat glands...................... 52

swelling... 14, 15, 18, 24, 30, 42, 46, 53, 64, 67, 68, 70, 72, 73, 98, 102, 125, 129, 148, 186

symptoms.. 8, 10, 14, 18, 34, 40, 43, 60, 63, 70, 74, 78, 87, 90, 91, 97, 102, 105, 108, 126, 128, 129, 142, 145, 198, 201, 206, 213

synergistically .. 94, 124, 200

synthetic 38, 61, 67, 93, 107, 109, 112, 158, 162, 184, 196

tap water.................. 133, 134

tendonitis......................... 120

tendons...................... 11, 145

thiamine 85

Thyroid 35, 36

tissue condition 79

tissues.. 40, 44, 78, 119, 121, 143, 147, 182, 197

tobacco companies 193, 195, 208, 216, 221

toxic. 44, 47, 52, 72, 94, 108, 111, 121, 122, 134, 182, 186, 188, 192, 193, 196, 197, 215, 221

toxins. 43, 46, 51, 52, 53, 68, 69, 71, 75, 78, 91, 95, 109, 118, 119, 120, 121, 129, 131, 137, 141, 159, 192

trace elements........... 49, 107

tuberculosis 28

Turkey 38

ulcers...... 161, 211, 212, 214

uric acid............. 97, 98, 170

varicose veins................. 107

vegetable oils ... 39, 167, 173

vegetables...... 28, 39, 48, 50, 103, 104, 139, 169, 170, 181, 185, 188, 189

virus.............. 43, 53, 66, 200

vitamin A 85

Vitamin B$_{12}$ 35

vitamin B$_6$ 94

vitamin B-6 85

vitamin C. 85, 106, 111, 112, 124, 157, 194, 219, 221

vitamin C flush............... 124

vitamin E. 68, 106, 112, 113, 114, 119, 120, 163, 219

vitamins8, 49, 62, 82, 92, 93, 94, 95, 96, 103, 112, 113, 131, 132, 155, 157, 159, 162, 163, 182, 184, 186, 199, 200, 202, 204, 205, 214, 215, 218, 221

water-soluble............ 96, 132

weight 11, 19, 23, 45, 50, 89, 107, 132, 145, 169, 183

Wheat 38, 162, 166

wheelchair 9, 51, 126, 217

white blood cells . 42, 52, 76, 77, 79

white flour 98, 154, 163, 230

white rice 163

white willow bark 70, 85

whole-wheat ... 163, 169, 186

x-rays 20, 21

yucca 71, 85

zinc 85, 94, 163, 189

CPSIA information can be obtained at www.ICGtesting.com
Printed in the USA
268549BV00002B/374/A